HEART MAFIA

HEART MAFIA

Bold Exposure of the Shameful Truth of India's Celebrated Cardiologists

Dr. Biswaroop Roy Chowdhury

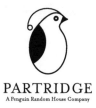

PARTRIDGE
A Penguin Random House Company

To order additional copies of this book, contact
Partridge India
000 800 10062 62
orders.india@partridgepublishing.com

www.partridgepublishing.com/india

Contents

Stop !

If you are about to gobble your routine diabetes pill or blood pressure or cholesterol lowering drug or going to inject an insulin shot!

or

If you are in a doctor's chamber and about to sign a consent form for angiography, bypass surgery or angioplasty

Then Stop !

Take an hour and finish reading this book. I understand you may be having many important tasks in hand which may force you to postpone reading the book. But remember the most important thing in your life is your life itself.

I bet after reading the next 100 pages you will never be able to see the medical industry with the same respect as you are having till now. Rather you will feel your current health condition is a trap by medical industry just for profit. The knowledge in the next few pages will help you to come out of the trap of drug dependency and life threatening surgeries and will guide you towards a lifelong good health.

I have written this book for the one and only cause i.e. 'Your Health—the Nation's Health' even though it may mean inviting lots of criticism and threat from profit minded medical fraternity. Help me in spreading this life saving knowledge by distributing this book among your friends and loved ones.

Get in touch with me at:
E-mail:biswaroop@yahoo.com

Face-book:
www.facebook.com/biswaroop-Roy-Chowdhury

Twitter:
https://twitter.com/biswarooproy

Linkedin:
www.linkedin.com/pub/dr-biswaroop-roy-chowdhury/
58/618/866

Wishing you the best of health.

Dr. Biswaroop Roy Chowdhury

Comment on 'Heart Mafia'

"Heart Mafia gives vivid picture of the exploitations of the patients by the cardiologists and heart surgeons. We need a radical change in the treatment of heart disease towards non invasive care. I congratulate Dr. Biswaroop Roy 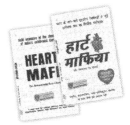 Chowdhury for the bold step of publishing this book.**

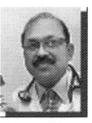

Dr Bimal Chajjer MBBS MD,
EX-Cardiac Physiacian
(AIIMS—New Delhi)
Heart Care and Lifestyle Expert,
Saaol Heart Center
(www.Saaol.com)

"I have a firm belief that the people suffering from heart-diseases and common masses who are determined not to be fooled and exploited by greedy persons within medical industry, will greatly benefit by this 'must-read' book!"

-Raj Rup Fuliya (IAS)
Additional Chief Secretary
Haryana Government, Chandigarh

"'Heart Mafia' is a bold book and it has true potential to change the manner medical science is practiced in India."

-Dr. Brij Bhushan Goel
(Naturopathy & Yoga)
All India Nature Cure Federation

Comment on
'How to Return from the Hospital Alive'

"I congratulate Dr Biswaroop for bringing out the true picture of pharmaceutical industry. We recommend health education as a part of regular school curriculum so that children understand that Good Health is their Birth 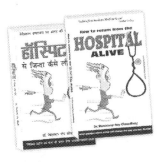 Right. They should also understand that only nature and natural products can ensure good health life long."

-Dr. Bharti Gandhi,
Director-Founder City
Montessori School, Lucknow
(World's Largest School—
Guinness World Records—2013)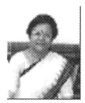

"I certainly appreciate this book. It is interesting, important and should be distributed"

-Dr. T. Colin Campbell
(Bill Clinton's Doctor)
Chief Scientist—The China Study

Research & Development Head : Rachna Sharma
Research & Development Team : Pratiksha Vats, Dr. Indupreet
Editing   : Rachna Sharma
Proofreading   : Neelam Kapoor, Pratiksha Vats,
                              Manmohan Rawat, Apeerna S

Graphics Designing   : Shankar Singh Koranga
Marketing   : Mohan Joshi
Music Director/composer   : Atul Swami
Singer   : Purnima, Abhijeet, Sunil
                              Thakur, Atul
Screenplay   : Minakshi, Atul
Animator   : Prakash
Link for song: www.indiabookofrecords.in/heartmafiasong

Edition   : January 2014
Published By   : Idea Publication
                              B-121, 2nd Floor, Green Fields,
                              Faridabad-121010(Haryana)
Phone   : +91 129 2510534,
                              +91 9312286540
Website   : www.biswaroop.com
Email   : biswaroop@yahoo.com
                              facebook: www.facebook.com/
                              heartmafia.official

Twitter: https:
//twitter.com/biswarooproy

Linkedin:
www.linkedin.com/pub/dr-biswaroop-roy-chowdhury/58/618/866

DEDICATION

Dedicated to my parents who have been the source
of inspiration for my investigative journalism.

Foreword

Dr. Bimal Chhajer MBBS, MD
Ex Cardic Physician (AIIMS—New Delhi)
Heart Care and Lifestyle Expert
Saaol Heart Center
(www.Saaol.com)

The cardiologists, interventional cardiologists and the heart surgeons have been exploiting the heart patients for the past few decades to make money—this is a simple fact that cannot be denied at all. Instead of telling the patients what leads to a heart disease, what they should do so that the blocks do not come up and what kind of food they should take to stop or reverse the disease, they are operating on these unfortunate heart patients or putting them on anti angina medicines.

The proof of the above statement lies in the fact that the number of heart patients has increased and so is the number of deaths due to heart attack. The doctors have failed to control this disease. In contrast, the number of small Pox patients has become zero and the Polio patients are almost nonexistent. In one the cause of the disease was removed and in the other case, the cause was not at all removed. The heart disease kept on increasing. The cardiologists and the heart surgeons are earning huge amount of money, heart hospitals have come up in every city in large number. It is a simple case of conspiracy. Patients' lack of knowledge about the cause of the blockages has become a boon for these money-spinning heart doctors.

It is an open secret. People worry about heart attacks and deaths. They do not want to have heart attacks, but they do not know how a heart attack takes place. They are unaware of the fact that heart attack cannot take place if the growth of the heart blockages stopped or reversed. When the heart patients reach heart hospitals, the interventional cardiologists (those who perform angiography and put stents) and the heart surgeons (those who perform bypass surgery) create a fear psychosis that heart attack is just one minute away. In the panic response, most of the patients and their relatives agree for a heart operation and end up paying the savings of their whole life. This is, in simple terms, the modus operandi of the Heart Mafia.

This unethical practice cannot go on for a long time. Someone has to protest; someone has to take a bold step. This is what Dr. Biswaroop has done through this book. He has not only substantiated his stand by giving facts and figures about the exploitations of the heart patients, but he has also highlighted the solutions though his book. He has got unique opportunity to work with 'The China Study' group where he has got very good exposure about heart care. Being simple and cheaper, Dr. Biswaroop's remedies are applicable to all the common people desirous of preventing heart disease.

I congratulate him for the eye opening book.

Chapter 1

DARD–E–DIL—
The Broken Heart

Nothing in this world can destroy your happiness more than trying to live with an illness, or a chronic sickness.

If you are a stent holder (angioplasty), or have undergone coronary bypass surgery, or on cholesterol lowering drug for quite some time or struggling to control your blood sugar with medication or on hypertension lowering drugs for some years and suddenly you come to know that you never needed those medical procedures and medications and that you are trapped in a conspiracy just for profit and may even get killed not because of the sickness but of the modern therapy. I am well aware that it's a very serious allegation on the medical fraternity in general and reputed cardiologists in particular.

But before you conclude anything, take a look at the below mentioned case of some Mr. B.

Mr. B. at the age of 58 had to undergo four-vessel coronary bypass grafting in Sept 2,2004. In 2005 he underwent an emergency pleural (lungs) effusion surgery.

Later on Feb 11, 2010, he underwent 2 coronary stent implantations (angioplasties) and by 2011 he was a person on death bed, after all these medical procedures his body mass increased by few kilos and the brain mass reduced by few units. He then came across the 'China Study Diet' or 'Whole Food Plant Based Diet' (WFPB)' and decided to follow the diet for six months even though not very strictly. As a result within six months his clogged arteries cleaned up, calcium deposits washed away, stent got cleared, weight reduced to normal and he became an active energetic and charismatic man as he was while he was the president of USA. In August 2011 in an exclusive interview to CNN, Mr. Bill Clinton disclosed the secrets of his recovery by stating:—

> "I did it because after I had these stents put in, I realized that, even though it happens quite often after you have bypasses because you lose the veins; the truth is that it clogged up, which meant the cholesterol was still causing build up in my vein that was part of my bypass. And I didn't want that to happen again."

So I did some research and found out that 82 percent of people since 1986 who had gone on a plant-based diet had begun to heal themselves; their arterial blockage cleared up, the calcium deposits around the heart broke. This movement was led by Dr. T. Colin Campbell of 'The China Study'. We now have 25 years of evidence and so I thought I'll become a part of this experiment and experience this self cleansing mechanism." Ultimately, Clinton said he wanted to be around to be a grandfather, and that was the major driving factor to follow the China Study Diet Plan. "That's really a big deal," he said. "Hillary and I, we're happy. We love our son-in-law. And if there's gonna be grandkids we wanna be around to do our part."

It was very clear from his interview that bypass surgery and angioplasty made his health rather worse. And finally it was 'The China Study Diet Plan' which helped him to revive his health. However this is not an exclusive example.

Let's take an example of another Mr. B.

At the age of 4 in 1977, he was diagnosed with a hole in his heart. The doctors recommended an open heart surgery to fill the hole. Although the surgeons were apparently able to fill the hole and fixed the problem but warned the boy's parents saying that the boy's heart will continue to remain weak throughout his life and he should refrain from any strenuous physical activity and sports. The boy with restricted physical activity and active sports passed through his school and college life.

In 2005, he discovered that the power of heart can be regained through certain kind of diet and lifestyle modification. He put himself on this diet and lifestyle modification regime called "The China Study Diet" for 2 years. In 2007 he put his heart on test by breaking a Guinness World Record for most number of push-ups in one minute (138 push-ups in 1 minute) by Roy Berger of Canada and creating a new record of 198 push-ups in 1 minute.

You must be wondering who this 2nd Mr. B is! This Mr. B. of course is not among 0.001% high profile people of the society, rather he belongs to the rest of the 99.999% of the common people living on this planet. Yet by now you know him little bit. After all you are reading a book written by him. He is Dr. Biswaroop Roy Chowdhury. It's me friends! Even now when I stand in front of the mirror and look at my deep long scar due to open heart surgery in my childhood on my chest the thought disturbs me "Had I known about the real healing power of the human body through diet and lifestyle that time, it would have been a better, playful and enjoyable childhood for me."

I took a formal training on 'The China Study Diet' from the chief scientist of 'The China Study', Dr. T. Colin Campbell, of Cornell University, who is also credited for the revival of Mr. Bill Clinton's Health.

However Dr T. Colin Campbell is neither the first doctor nor is it for the first time proven that no matter how worse the condition of your heart or severity of the disease is, you still can reverse the condition of your heart or even clear more than 95% blockage without any risky surgery and lifelong medication, just by following a special nutritional diet plan. This stands true for diabetes or high B.P or high cholesterol. All these conditions can be reversed through this nutritional plan.

Two cardiologists, Lester Morrison and John W. Gofman (almost 70 years ago) undertook studies in the 1940s and 1950s to determine the effect of diet on the people who already had a heart attack. The doctors put these patients on a special diet (similar to The China Study Diet) regime and found that the special diet dramatically reduced the subsequent recurrence of heart attacks/disease. Dr. Nathan Pritikin did the same thing in 1960s and 1970s. Then Dr. Caldwell Esselstyn (of Cleveland Clinic) and Dr. Dean Ornish set out to learn more in 1980s and 1990s. Working separately they both proved that the special diet can control and even reverse advanced heart diseases.

Besides Dr T. Colin Campbell, I got the opportunity to learn from Dr. Caldwell Esselstyn also.

I applied the knowledge of 'The China Study Diet Plan' to approximately 10,000 patients across 25 cities including Abu Dhabi, Dubai, Kuwait, Hanoi, Port-Bair, Sikkim, Siliguri, Hyderabad, Bangalore, Faridabad, Vapi, Jaipur, Lucknow, Tumkur, Bhilwara, Almora, Shimla, Agartala, Pune, Chandigarh, Bhopal, Nagpur, Satara, Rajkot, Mysore, Kota etc.. Among them the prominent ones are my health training with Indian Army last year (2013) in Port Blair (where 800 jawans participated in the training but only 180 agreed to follow the prescribed diet plan) and a health workshop with Haryana Govt. Teachers (250 in number).

I must tell you that whether it is a participant in one of my health workshops or a patient in my Faridabad Clinic I am yet to meet a single patient who has followed "The China Study Diet Plan" and has not benefitted and reversed his heart disease.

Now the obvious question is, if a person can get cured just by putting himself on a specific diet (The China Study Diet) then why heart disease is the number one killer in the world! Why life threatening procedures like bypass surgery or angioplasty or expensive medication for diabetes, cholesterol or high B.P that are full of severe side effects, are flourishing so much that in most of the hospitals about 40% of the total revenue comes from the cardiology department.

The answer to this question is a clear cut profit motive.

Forget about the risks involved in bypass surgery or angioplasty, even the diagnosis of heart blockage is so risky that in India the total number of patients dying of angiography on the diagnosis table every year equals to the total number of people killed in all the terrorist attacks bomb blasts put together from 1987 to 2013.

Please note that people don't die of the heart diseases. More often patients die of the complications of the surgery and the long term side effects of the medication involved.

I would rather say the Indian cardiologists are suffering from "Oculostenotic Reflex Syndrome" a term to describe cardiologists who rush to intervene every single patient having heart blockage with angioplasty or a bypass surgery.

Humans are the only animals who die more often of the complications of heart (more so because of unnecessary and profit making medical interventions). Have you ever heard of a cat dying of a heart attack? Spontaneous heart attacks in non human mammals are exceedingly rare. In 1959 researchers at Northwestern University succeeded at inducing a heart attack in a laboratory animal. They were surprisingly frank about the rigors of this twelve year project. They had imported fifteen rhesus monkeys from India and fed a diet of monkey chow mixed with cholesterol butter suspended in water and bread soaked in cream. They lost several monkeys to fulminant tuberculosis, which swept through the animal lab. The monkeys, "completely undomesticable" ate only some of their food and threw the leftover around their cages. Some escaped from the cages.

The researchers spent hours chasing them as they swung among the hanging light fixtures. Years of frustrating work eventually paid off. One female monkey struggled mightily with the researchers as they removed her from her cage to photograph her. The strain was too much, half an hour later, she collapsed and died. When the researchers performed the autopsy, they saw three thrombotic occlusions and a massive myocardial infarction. They concluded that they had achieved the first heart attack in an experimental animal. Something (heart attack) which is nearly impossible in animals is so common in humans that every third death in the developing & developed countries is because of heart disease and India is leading with 60% of the world's heart patients being Indians (WHO estimate).

The area (and shape) of each of the country in the figure given in next page is morphed so that the size is proportional to the number of deaths due to heart attack in a particular country.

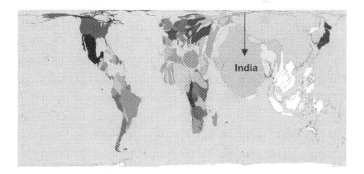

Little surprise that in India cardiology is the most profitable business with more than 400 heart hospitals. Half of which are located in six cities only.

Through this book I challenge all Indian cardiologists and cardiac surgeons to prove that the procedures like angioplasty and bypass surgery are not only life threatening but also have no evidence of extending the life or improving the quality of life of a patient and are just profit driven procedures. But I also know that people (cardiologists) who have built their career and fortune upon these procedures (angioplasty and bypass surgery) can act like threatened dictators. They want to cling to the power at all costs, and the more they are challenged, the nastier and dangerous they become. I would like to conclude this chapter by highlighting an obsolete paradigm that reigned for hundreds of years: the idea that the sun revolves around the earth and not the other way. When Copernicus published **De Revolutionibus Orbium Coelestium 1543** asserting that the earth revolved around the sun, he was challenging common sense, a millennium of scientific agreement and an outraged religious community. The fact that he had evidence—that his theory is a fact explained phenomenon that were earlier unexplainable under the prevailing earth centric theory didn't matter a bit. Likewise the stark truth exposed in this book will be vehemently denied by some (those with a profit motive) and will not be accepted. As a philosopher-songwriter Paul Frederic Simon puts it,

"A man hears what he wants to hear and disregards the rest".

Chapter 2

Heart Failure Mechanism

Imagine your heart as the central warehouse of a nationwide delivery system. The trucking fleet is your blood, ferrying vital supplies (oxygen and nutrients) to all corners of your body and picking up waste. Your arteries and veins are superhighways and secondary roads connecting cities and towns (cells and tissues) along the way. When the system is operating at prime efficiency, a steady stream of cargo-laden vehicles leaves the hub at a rapid clip every day. Once their freight is delivered, they return promptly to pick up the next load.

But contemplate for a minute what would happen if the dispatching operation faltered. Freight-filled trucks would jam the cargo bays. Empty vehicles would be stranded in remote locations, unavailable to pick up new deliveries. Customers along the routes would struggle to survive without fresh supplies.

In short, this is what happens in heart failure. Disease, injury, and years of wear and tear take a toll on the heart's pumping ability. When this once-powerful muscle struggles to circulate blood efficiently, a cascade of physiological changes is set in motion.

Although the term "heart failure" conjures up a catastrophic vision of a suddenly silent heart, the condition is more aptly described as a gradual decline in the heart's ability to pump. Heart failure is not a disease per se. Instead, it is a set of diverse physical symptoms. In medical lingo, this collection of complaints is known as a syndrome. The underlying common denominator is the heart's inability to circulate blood adequately.

How the healthy heart works

Your heart contracts and relaxes approximately 100,000 times a day. Most of the time you don't think about this ceaseless rhythm—that is, until something goes wrong.

Your cardiovascular system comprises a complex network of channels that convey oxygen, nutrients and waste products to and away from your tissues and organs. Your heart is at the center of this system. This muscle, the size of two adult fists, propels a Herculean 2,000 gallons of blood daily. Extending from your heart is a web of blood vessels that reaches to the farthest corners of your body. Laid end to end, these vessels would stretch more than 60,000 miles. The vessels that transport oxygen-rich blood out from the heart are called the arteries; the veins return oxygen-depleted blood to the lungs and heart.

All the parts of the cardiovascular system—the heart's chambers, its electrical signaling center, valves, and blood vessels—work in concert to ensure that blood moves through the body efficiently. This level of complex organization demands precise timing and impeccable coordination. If any part of the sequence falters, the workings of the entire system are in jeopardy.

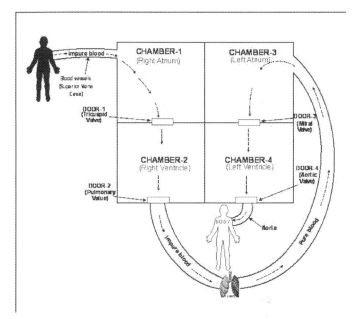

To understand the functioning of heart, imagine that the impure blood (deoxygenated blood) from the body enters the chamber-1 (right atrium) and through the Door-1 (Tricuspid Valve) to chamber 2 (right ventricle) through the pumping (squeezing) action of the walls of the chamber 1. From chamber-2 the oxygen deficient blood is pushed into the lungs through the Door-2 (Pulmonary valve), where it is filled with oxygen (CO_2 is exchanged with oxygen). The oxygen rich blood now travels from lung to Chamber-3 (left atrium) and then to Chamber-4 (left ventricle) through Door 3(Mitral Valve) by the pumping actions of the walls of the chambers. From here the blood is then sent back to the body through Door-4 (Aortic valve), so as to distribute the oxygen and nutrients to the body.

During the relaxed diastolic, phase, the atria (upper chambers) fill with blood. The walls of the atria then contract, pushing the blood through the valves into the relaxed ventricles (lower chambers). The valves close tightly during contractions to prevent the back flow of blood. When the ventricles have filled, the systolic phase of the heart cycle occurs, in which the ventricle walls compress powerfully to expel the blood out of the heart and into the arteries. The entire sequence is masterminded by a group of cells in the wall of the right atrium called the sinoatrial (SA) node. This structure emits tiny electrical impulses that signal the heart chambers when to contract. Because the SA node determines the heart's pace and rhythm, it is sometimes called your natural pacemaker.

What happens in heart failure

Heart failure may start with injury from a heart attack, develop as a result of damaged valves, or be brought on by an infection or a disease. Many times, it is the product of years of toil against high blood pressure and clogged blood vessels (arteries). Regardless of exactly what sets the process in motion, heart failure culminates in a progressive weakening of your heart's power to pump. Consequently, blood circulates through your heart and body more slowly; your cells thirst for fresh oxygen and nutrients.

Outward signs of the cardiac muscle's subpar performance may remain hidden for months or even years while heart failure advances. To compensate for its weakened state, the heart undergoes a series of structural transformations known as cardiac remodeling. In an effort to expel blood more forcefully, the walls of the left heart chamber thicken, or the chamber may dilate and take on a rounder shape, which allows it to hold a larger quantity of blood.

Other physical processes also come to the heart's aid as it struggles to maintain sufficient output. Levels of stress hormones, which signal the heart to beat faster and harder in times of need, rise. Blood vessels constrict in an effort to keep blood pressure stable despite the fact that a lower quantity of blood is being pumped out. Circulation is also diverted away from the skin and less important tissues so that the heart and brain receive a steady supply of oxygen and nutrients. In turn the diminished blood flow to the kidneys activates a set of hormones that prompt the body to retain sodium and fluid in an attempt to supplement the total volume of circulating blood.

In the short run, these fixes enable the heart to deliver a near-normal level of blood to the tissues. But the solution is only temporary. Ultimately, these alterations hasten the heart's decline. The heart's modified shape increases the stress on the muscle as it attempts to consume more oxygen. Eventually, the benefits obtained from this accelerated pumping diminish. The faster heartbeat and narrowed blood vessels amplify the heart's workload, and the costs of the additional yield outweigh the advantages of increased output.

Symptoms of heart failure

Heart failure generates two major obstacles for the body: (1) the tissues and organs don't get enough oxy gen, and (2) fluid builds up in the lungs and tissues. Each of these problems spawns a series of distinct complaints. If you're unfamiliar with heart failure, you could easily interpret these as isolated symptoms. Doctors and patients alike frequently attribute early signs of heart failure to poor physical fitness, overweight, or just "getting old." The clinical picture is further clouded by the fact that these manifestations can come and go and get better or worse over the course of the illness.

Mental confusion: The brain doesn't get enough oxygen

Weight gain: The buildup of excess fluid causes an increase in body weight.

Fatigue: Less blood reaches the working muscles.

Skin changes: Blood flow is diverted to vital organs, causing skin to feel cold and take on a bluish color.

Lung congestion: Excess fluid backs up from the heart into the lungs.

Shortness of breath: Fluid in the lungs causes breathing difficulties, especially during exertion or when lying down.

Coughing and wheezing: Fluid in the lungs causes these problems, too.

Loss of appetite: The accumulation of fluid in the liver and stomach leads to feelings of nausea.

Swelling (feet, legs, abdomen): Excess fluid settles in tissues.

What causes heart failure?

The defining characteristic of heart failure is a mal-functioning cardiac muscle. But many different circumstances can lead to this end point. Sometimes the origin of heart failure lies in mechanical defects of the muscle itself that can be present from birth or brought on by disease or events later in life. Heart failure can also evolve from conditions that habitually overwork the heart, eventually wearing it out. Often, multiple factors are at the root of heart failure. The following are some of the more common causes of heart failure.

Coronary artery disease. Approximately two out of three cases of heart failure can be traced to coronary artery disease, the narrowing of the blood vessels (arteries) that feed the heart muscle cells. When cholesterol-laden deposits form on the inside walls of the arteries, there's less space available for blood flow. The lack of adequate oxygen leaves the heart muscle starved for blood. Coronary artery disease also sets the stage for heart muscle damage from a heart attack, another cause of heart failure.

- **Dead or dying heart tissue.** When one of the fatty deposits on the inside of the artery wall bursts open, the blood forms a clot, much the way the body would respond if you cut your finger. If a clot forms in one of the arteries that feed the heart muscle, it can cut off the flow of oxygen to the tissue that lies beyond the clot. This sudden stopping of blood flow to part of the heart muscle is called a myocardial infarction, or heart attack. In the aftermath of a nonfatal heart attack, heart tissue may be seriously damaged or dead, depending on how long blood flow was interrupted. The patches of compromised tissue may not be able to beat with the force needed to push blood through the body. Approximately a quarter of people who survive a heart attack develop heart failure within the next year.

- **High blood pressure (hypertension).** Blood pressure is a measure of the force it takes to move blood through the vessels. The higher the pressure, the harder the heart must work. Just as the muscles in your arms buildup when you lift weights, the heart muscle thickens in response to pumping against extra resistance. Instead of strengthening the heart, however, this bulking up does just the opposite. The thickened muscle consumes more oxygen. It also can't fully relax between contractions. The net effect is that the heart muscle gradually stops beating as forcefully as it should. High blood pressure precedes heart failure in 75% of cases.

- **Cardiomyopathy.** This is an umbrella term used to describe a number of diseases that result from damage to the heart muscle.

- **Dilated cardiomyopathy**. By far the most common form of the condition, this type of cardiomyopthy is characterized by stretching and thinning of the ventricle walls. It can be brought on by a viral or bacterial infection or develop from long-term exposure to alcohol, cocaine, or other toxins. There is also growing evidence that inherited forms of the disorder result from specific chromosome defects.

- **Hypertrophic cardiomyopathy.** This inherited disorder usually appears in young adulthood and is more common in men than in women. It causes an extreme thickening of the ventricle wall.
- **Restrictive cardiomyopathy.** In this condition, the heart muscle becomes extremely stiff, which prevents it from filling with blood properly. The pumping phase of the heart cycle is initially unaffected.

Sometimes, restrictive cardiomyopathy stems from conditions that cause scarring of the heart muscle or the formation of deposits of iron or certain proteins in the cardiac cells. In other cases, the origin is unknown.

- **Heart valve damage.** Faulty heart valves that don't open or close efficiently put additional strain on the heart. Disease, infection, heart attack, and aging can all cause damage to the valves. When a valve is narrowed, or stenotic, it doesn't open completely to let blood pass from the chamber. This causes pressure to build up in the heart. A leaky valve allows blood to travel backward between beats, forcing the heart to do double duty to keep blood moving forward.
- **Diabetes.** Over time, uncontrolled diabetes weakens the heart muscle by causing coronary artery disease (a major risk factor for heart failure) and damage to the kidneys.
- **Heart rhythm disturbances.** An abnormally fast heartbeat can produce structural changes in the heart's left ventricle.

Chapter 3

Jiyo ji Bhar Ke
The Illusion of Nutrition
Supplements

Whenever a patient is diagnosed with any health ailment whether it is diabetes or high B.P or high cholesterol or heart disease or even a case of obesity; doctors along with the medication are quick to add some kind of nutritional supplements and multivitamin tablets. Whether you are consuming nutritional supplements or tonics recommended by doctors or you are taking multivitamin capsules or milk powder or protein supplements on your own just for general wellbeing, you must understand that consuming such nutritional products are not just waste but even injurious to health.

The title of this chapter "Jiyo Ji Bhar Ke" must be reminding you of a very frequent commercial advertisement in every major T.V Channel and newspaper of Revital—a multivitamin supplement. Salman Khan being the present brand ambassador for the advertisement claims that not only is he consuming Revital for the last 15 years which is the major contributor of his great body but also his father had been consuming it for a very long time. Yuvraj Singh, the previous brand ambassador of Revital was dropped suddenly for the obvious reason (immediately after being diagnosed with cancer). Even though we may not trust the T.V commercial literally but this fact is also true that nutritional supplement business have been growing by leaps and bounds in the last 10 years. Let's have a second look at how the nutritional supplements work in our body and also in your mind (the belief that it works).

Let's start with an imaginary situation in which one of your acquaintance is recently diagnosed with diabetes and the doctor has advised him to refrain from sugar. Now think for a while, what alternative comes in your mind to replace sugar? I know for most of us it will be sugar free. Now try to recall your memory and find how you acquired this information that for diabetics, sugar can be replaced with so called healthy sugar free. Was it mentioned in any text book or was it recommended by a doctor?

What you will recall is the commercial T.V advertisement with Bipasha Basu flaunting—"Meri-figure Ka Raj Hai—Sugar free". How reliable is this advertisement or for that matter Bipasha Basu? Is she a doctor or a scientist?

Let's go back a little into the history to know the origin of sugar free. In 1964, the chief chemist of G.D. Searle & Company accidently tasted a chemical called 'aspartame' which happened to be 10 times sweeter than sugar and upon analysis found to be 20 times cheaper than the commercially available sugar. It made a good business sense. They planned to mass produce it for commercial sale for human consumption. So they applied to FDA (Food and Drug Administration) for a No-Objection certificate for human consumption. Upon research and analysis. FDA found that aspartame (now called as sugar free) may lead to more than 150 diseases including diabetes, heart disease, high cholesterol, high B.P, obesity etc. FDA didn't approve aspartame for mass production. But G.D. Searle & Company was determined about this commercial endeavor so they persuaded the case in the court in 1982. Then the newly appointed FDA commissioner, Arthur Hayes Hull Jr. approved the chemical aspartame for human consumption. Later it was discovered that Arthur Hayes Hull, Jr was having financial ties with G.D. Searle & Company. Arthur was sacked from FDA and he promptly joined G.D. Searle & Company as a P.R Manager. However by this time the sugar free syndrome had penetrated so deep and spread so wide that it could not be banned for human consumption although several attempts were made to do so. So forget about diabetic patients, even if a healthy person consumes sugar free products for a few months, he may develop diabetes. Sugar free is more harmful than the conventional refined sugar. At this point we need to understand why anything refined like sugar, salt, refined oil or products made up of refined material like biscuits, chips or various kinds of packed/processed/fast food are harmful.

Let's say you are consuming sugar through tea. To absorb and metabolize this sugar the body needs minerals like chromium, manganese, cobalt, zinc and magnesium. Though these minerals are already present in sugarcane juice and beetroot juice from which sugar is derived; these minerals get discarded during the refining process of sugar. This means to absorb and utilize sugar for energy, body is dependent on its own reserve of the above said minerals. But this reserve will not last long and will get exhausted as you are consuming too many sugary and other refined products. It will lead to various illnesses including heart disease and high B.P.

Deficiency of various minerals and vitamins may lead to a number of conditions like low immunity, constant fatigue, body ache, frequent cough and cold, loss of weight or obesity, which may force you to visit your local physician. The doctor upon diagnosing some vitamin and mineral deficiency will prescribe you a multivitamin pill to recover this deficiency, but the mechanism of multivitamin pills itself is faulty.

Let's say you are prescribed a Vitamin C tablets to recover from vitamin C deficiency. But what this vitamin C tablet actually does to the body is shown in through this flowchart.

High Vitamin C intake ⟶ Copper deficiency

Poor Absorption & Utilization of Vitamin B1, Vitamin B2 Vitamin B6, Vitamin E ⟵ Iron Toxicity

⟶ Imbalance in the Bio-Chemistry of the body

Flavonoids 14-36 mg	Phosphorous 14.2mg
Biotin 0.95g	Potassium 109.7mg
Energy 48.cal	Zinc 0.06mg
Vitamin A RE 3.0g	Carbohydrate 10.7g
Vitamin K 3.3g	Unsaturated fat 0.09g

Manganese 4.6mg	Fluoride 0.01mg
Sugar 10.2g	Sucrose 2.36g
Mono-un saturated fat 0.009g	Poly-unsaturated fat 0.08g
A-Carotene 0.1g	Fructose 5.83g
Protein 0.3g	Fat 0.23g
Glucose 2.07g	Saturated Fat 0.02g
Total Dietary Fibre	2.16g Sodium 0.002g
Salt 0.005g	Starch 0.06g
Chloride 0.3mg	Calcium 5.0mg
Iron 0.17mg	Manganese 4.6mg
Copper 0.03mg	Selenium 0.16g
Chromium 0.76g	Molybdenum 0.1g
Iodine 0.5g	Vitamin C 5.6mg
Vitamin B1 0.02mg	Vitamin B2 0.02mg
Vitamin B3 0.14mg	Pantothenic acid 0.04mg
Vitamin B6 0.05mg	Folate 2.78g
Choline 3.4mg	Vitamin E 0.45mg
Trans fat 0	Cholesterol 0
B-Carotene 13.6g	B-Cryptoxanthin 12.4g
Lycopene 0g	Lutein & xeaxanthin 27.8g
Phytosterols 15.3mg	Water 84.3ml
Pectin 0.5g (may vary)	

You will observe that all the nutrients are in a very delicate balance in such a manner that when you consume an apple as a whole, all the above nutrients react with each other to make a perfect balance so as to get absorbed and utilized by the body without disturbing the homeostasis (inner balance) of the body. The intricate calculation of the combination of nutrients while packaging fruits/vegetables can be achieved only by nature. This calculation is beyond the comprehension of humans. There are 4 elements within a naturally occurring whole food supplement that are not analyzed by most scientists. They are Hormones, Oxygen content, Phytochemicals and Enzymes i.e. H.O.P.E.

Here: I find the folding umbrella analogy appropriate. The nutrients trapped inside the fruits and vegetables (before cooking/processing) can be compared with an open foldable umbrella. Once it enters your body it can get squeezed (fold) and sneak inside the cells of the body and again can open and become active. However once the nutrient is extracted from the fruits/vegetables and converted into a pill/powder/tonic in isolated form it loses its capability to the change shape and remain just an open umbrella structurally similar to the original nutrients but functionally may not be so absorbable by the body.

To make you understand the complex mechanism in a simplified form. I will share with you an explanation which I came across while attending one of the lectures by Dr. T. Colin Campbell, in Cornell University.

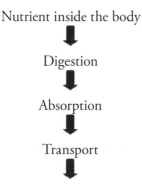

Nutrient inside the body

⬇

Digestion

⬇

Absorption

⬇

Transport

⬇

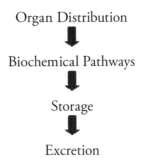

Organ Distribution

Biochemical Pathways

Storage

Excretion

When we consume a nutrient, the first thing that happens is that it has to be digested. What I am thinking about in this case, (in the course of digestion in the intestine), is the extent to which the nutrient is released from its food as a single nutrient floating around ready to do something. So, the extent to which the nutrient in the food is actually digested and extracted for subsequent absorption, the percentage that is actually digested can vary quite substantially, maybe from, (in some cases), nearly 0% at times to as high as 30% or 40%, 50%. So, we have a big variation in digestibility of a given nutrient.

Then it's absorbed across the intestinal wall and here again, we already know the mechanisms that control the percentage of a nutrient that crosses the intestinal wall—that gets into the bloodstream. And some of the finer details of that have already been published, have been examined for years-decades, even—and it's very intricate process. But the body is always capable of determining at any point in time what percentage of the nutrient that has been digested is actually absorbed. So now we have two levels of variation. First, the percent that's digested. Second, the percent that is actually absorbed is itself a fraction of the proportion that was digested. This percent of a percent can vary (according to) all sorts of different factors, especially those factors that are in the immediate environment that may relate to pH, or other physical-chemical effects.

Now it's in the blood and it's carried through the blood—'transported'. And some of these nutrients, especially the lipid-soluble nutrients, are now transported on little carriers in the blood—maybe protein carriers for example. Beta-Carotene, just to give an example, is carried on LDL protein particles. The activity of those nutrients at any point in time is going to be greatly influenced by the percent that's actually on the carrier as opposed to the percent that is not on the carrier. The percent that is actually carried on these carriers varies, and when it's bound to the carrier it's generally considered to be inactive. When it's free, floating around, it's considered to be more active. So the percent that's bound to the carrier compared to the percent that's not, can vary. And so once again, we see that this variation in the utilization of nutrients in food occurs at many levels in the digestion and metabolism process. At each stage, the percentage of nutrients that passes on to the next stage is adjusted.

So now we can think about another process, having to do with how much of the nutrient is distributed to different organs. It may want to go to the liver, to the pancreas, to the lung, whatever. Or to the bone and so the body is determining in its own intricate, really fascinating ways, how much of the nutrient is going to be deliverable to different organs. And again, this can vary quite substantially. And if you think of all this variation that can occur from digestion to organ distribution, that's almost nothing compared to the variation that occurs once it's inside the cell and then is metabolized to various and sundry metabolites. These are the very intricate biochemical pathways that exist for a lot of different nutrients, and there are so many pathways that a nutrient can take in so far as the formation of metabolites and products, each of which are being, produced for some special purpose. May be they are going to actually function at the site that needs some activity. Maybe they are going to be distributed to some place where they are going to be stored. Possibly they might be, as we say sometimes, deactivated or detoxified and then excreted. Again, this is highly variable thing that is changing on a minute-by-minute basis, even on a microsecond-by microsecond basis.

This means in one meal you consume 100 milligram of vitamin C and 400 milligram of vitamin C in another meal? Does it mean that in the second meal your body has absorbed and utilized 4 times the Vitamin C in comparison to the first meal? Certainly not. It is impossible to calculate how much amount of nutrients your body is going to utilize after consuming a particular multivitamin pill.

To understand it further consider the 1999 Noble Prize Winning Research work by Dr Guntur Blobel. He found that proteins posses inherent signals or information that determine which cells attract and absorb them and where in the cells the protein belong.

This finding about proteins opened a doorway for intercellular chemical research that provides us with a principle that has applications for the issue of synthetic and natural nutrients. Nutrients do not simply wander around inside the human body in search of a nutrient poor cell to colonize. Instead, it is as if nutrients contain address and zip codes that enable them to be delivered directly to cells containing the same addresses and zip codes. This is nature's postal system within the body and synthetic nutrients isolated in laboratories cannot match the simplicity and effectiveness of that system. It is a system that helps to explain why natural nutrients in fruits and vegetables are much more absorbable and bio-available to us than synthetics.

That is the reason why it is well established that beta-carotene in fruits and vegetables taken in raw form protect against lung cancer whereas beta-carotene in pill form known to promote lung cancer. Same is true for other nutrients. For example copper when consumed as a part of the whole vegetable is known to keep cholesterol down whereas copper in supplements or synthetic form is known to increase the risk of mortality by 5.9 % (BBC-2003).

All kinds of baby food and milk powder comes under supplement categories.

According to 'The China Study':

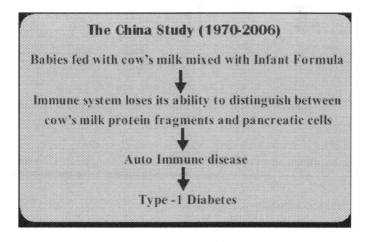

In March 2012 Supreme Court of India issued a notice to Bournvita, Horlicks, Maltova, Complan, Mylo, Boost, Pediasure, HR Pro, Maxi Nutrition (protein milk) etc. for their misleading advertisement.

Similarly F.D.A (U.S.A) has issued a permanent injunction forbidding Nutralite from making unsubstantiated claims.

By now you have seen ample evidences that the consumption of multivitamin pills, tonics, health/protein powder are useless and severely injurious to health.

But your long held belief that consumption of vitamin pills and supplement powder contributes greatly to your health may be stopping you to accept the above scientific evidence.

Read the following example to re-consider your belief on multivitamins supplements, health tonics, and protein powder and milk products. Here at this point you may be confused thinking that at many occasions and many places including some reported journals you might have read that supplement consumption is good and necessary for health so as to overcome various deficiencies in the body. So whom to trust. The one which you have just read in this chapter or your long held belief about Food Supplements!

The answer is "Cochrane Report"—(Supreme Authority among Reports/Journals). Cochrane is a WHO recognized organization having branches in more than 100 countries including India (Vellore). One of their jobs is to collect all kinds of reports related to a particular research and make a final analysis of the outcome.

In March 14, 2012 Cochrane released a report where they have collected data related to "Whether consumption of Food Supplement is good or bad for health".

Cochrane Summaries

Independent High-quality evidence for health care decision making

Antioxidant Supplements for prevention of mortality in healthy participants and patients with various diseases.

Bjelakovic G, Nikolova D, Gluud LL, Simonetti RG, Gluud C Published Online March 14,2012

Conclusion: Vitamin and Mineral supplements increases the mortality in patients with various diseases and in general population as well.

Chapter 4

The Profitable Science of Heart Disease

What is the most important principle to make any business profitable? It's obvious answer . . . repeat customers! If the customers come back to you time and again for availing your services, your business may grow exponentially. This is the basis of the treatment of heart diseases, even if it is dangerous to the patient and may lead to death.

The journey of heart treatment starts with 'diagnosis' that often consists of several kinds of X-rays scans and invasive procedure like angiography. The moment you enter into a hospital with a discomfort, the easiest thing for the doctor is to order for various kinds of diagnostic tests. To start with is an x-ray or a CAT scan or CT scan etc. More so in the hospitals that boast of their latest diagnostic techniques; as reported in an article in Time Magazine called "The Hospital War". More often hospitals buy expensive scanning machines on loan basis and to meet the monthly installments of the machine they calculate the number of scans/patients per month required to make it to the installments. These number of patients (for diagnosis) become the unsaid target for the doctors. This act of hospitals become not only an unnecessary financial burden on patients but is also quite damaging to their body. For instance, a 64 slice whole body CAT scan provides 15.2 mSv of radiations for man and 21.4 mSv for women (women's denser body tissue and breast require higher doses to get clear image). Compare this number with the level of radiations to which the survivor of the atomic bomb explosion at Hiroshima and Nagasaki in Japan were exposed to an average dose between 5 mSv and 20 mSv with some doses as high as 50 mSv.

Since the radiation from all sources remain in our bodies throughout our life, the likelihood of average 21st century patients matching or even exceeding that average dose to which the population of Hiroshima and Nagasaki were exposed, is very high.

The other popular and profitable diagnostic method is Coronary Angiography. Here the cardiologist threads a catheter through the arteries of leg or arm or wrist, into the heart. They use a video monitor to see/conduct the whole procedure. Once the catheter reaches the blocked artery a dye is injected and the doctor takes a picture of the coronary artery (called a coronary angiography). The angiogram helps the doctor to see the size and location of the blockage or plaque. At this point we need to understand that the size of the blockage as estimated by the doctor is again illusive and totally depends upon the doctor's own approximation and guessing ability and varies substantially from cardiologist to cardiologist and that is not all about the procedure of angiography. Wire like object called catheter, while passing through the artery of various organs like kidney, liver, parts of intestine to its destination artery in heart, may cause damage to the organs leading to many permanent disabilities including death. If you go through the records of top hospitals like Safdarjung Hospital, G.B Pant Hospital and AIIMS you will notice that the death rates due to angiography are quite substantial. Approx 1% of angiographies that translate into number of deaths due to diagnostic procedure (angiography) every year equals 10 times the Indian soldiers that died during Kargil war. But these figures will not discourage a cardiologist from prescribing more angiographies because of the profitability factor and also the consent form has already been signed by the patients, where patient agrees that they understand that angiography may lead to death and they are ready for that. But in reality how many of the patients do you think might have read the consent form before signing? If you are lucky enough to pass through these deadly procedures safely, then comes the most interesting and most profitable procedures of all time—bypass surgery and angioplasty.

Through diagnostic angiography you will graduate to the knowledge that you are suffering from 70% or 80% or 90 % blockage of the arteries. etc. etc. etc.

But before that let's understand how the blockage occurred in the arteries in the first place. The innermost layer of a blood vessel is called endothelium. If all the endothelial cells of the body are laid out flat one cell thick they would be equivalent to 2 lawn tennis courts. Healthy blood vessels are strong and elastic. Their endothelial layer is smooth and unobstructed, allowing a free flow of blood. But when the level of fats in the bloodstream become elevated, everything begins to change. Gradually in the endothelium, white blood cells and platelets cause clotting. Cells become sticky. Eventually the white blood cells penetrate the endothelium, where they attempt to ingest the rising numbers of LDL (bad) cholesterol molecules. That are oxidized majorly from the fatty/processed diet. The white blood cells send out a call for help to other white blood cells. More and more of them get collected on the site and get stuck to bad cholesterol eventually forming a bubble of fatty pus-plaque. As they enlarge they severely narrow and sometimes block the arteries. A significantly narrowed artery cannot give the heart muscle, a normal blood supply. Thus deprivation causes chest pain or angina. However it is not the old larger plaque (70 % or more blockage) that puts you most at risk for heart attack. It is the small young plaque that ruptures at its outer lining or cap, and bleeds into the coronary artery.

As the plaque is formed, a fibrous cap develops at its top covered by a single layer of endothelium. For a while the protected plaque lies quietly in its place. Eventually the shearing force of blood flowing over the weakened cap may cause it to rupture. The plaque content now oozes out into the flowing bloodstream. To heal the ruptured area, the platelets become activated. They rush to the area and try to stop the invading garbage by clotting the rupture. The clot is self propagating and within minutes the entire artery may become blocked due to clot formation by platelets. With no more blood flowing through the blocked artery, heart muscles may die. This is the definition of heart attack.

More often the doctors equate the plaque accumulated overtime in the artery, like a deposit in the old pipes. As they grow they cause angina (pain) and eventually heart attack. Everyone has had this experience with the household plumbing. First a sink drains slowly and then one day it is so obstructed that it overflows. Many doctors and patients mapped the familiar and intuitive model of pipes into the problem of coronary artery disease.

The logic of therapeutic intervention here is clear. Arteries provide the network for blood flow. If the plaque obstruct flow in a patient with chronic angina, then plaque must be removed or the blood must be bypassed. Managing the plaque or unwanted deposits in this way would restore flow, reduce the frequency and severity of angina and prevent damage to the heart muscles. Such plumbing metaphors with all their intuitive appeal, were not simply a way describing and marketing angioplasty and bypass surgery to patients. They also influenced the thinking of the doctors powerfully.

But there is a missing link. One thing that differentiate the plaque deposits in human arteries and the blockage of the house sink is that in 87.5 % of the cases the cause of heart attacks is not the biggest plaque deposits in the arteries ranging from 70 % to 80 % or 90 % blockage but it is the smaller plaque like 30 % or 40% that are responsible for the heart attack as explained previously and managing these smaller plaques through angioplasty and bypass surgery is impossible because these are plenty in numbers.

Since the bypass surgery and angioplasty targets only the biggest plaque this means theoretically by removing the biggest plaque you are reducing the chances of further heart attacks only by 12.5%. But in reality it makes the patient's condition even more worse.

To understand why angioplasty and bypass surgery cannot improve the life expectancy of patient and rather increases the mortality (death rate). Let's understand how bypass surgery and angioplasty is done.

Look closely at the details of the bypass heart surgery. After an anesthetist renders the patient unconscious, the surgeon removes a portion of artery or veins called graft from the patient's arm or leg or chest. Then rib cage is cut open to stitch the bypass graft to the blocked coronary artery. Angioplasty involves only slightly less bravado. The cardiologist snakes a three foot long balloon tipped catheter into a coronary artery. The balloon ruptures the plaque, stretches the artery wall, and deploys a wire mesh stent to prop it open.

Now the problem with both the procedures is that the body somehow recognizes the surgery sites as dumping site and start pouring deposits and garbage within a few months and the artery again gets blocked.

According to the Archives of Internal Medicine (Medical Journal) Feb 2012, in a randomized trail 7229 patients who had undergone bypass surgery or angioplasty (between 1970 to 2011) were observed and compared with patients with similar severity of blockage but have not gone for surgery. The report concluded that no extra benefits are seen after surgery in patients in comparison to those who avoided surgery. Similar report was published in The New York Times (27 Feb 2012) also. Besides no benefit these surgeries come with many life long side effects. One of them is poor mental ability post surgery. Doctors stop the heart during surgery and the blood is rerouted through the heart lung machine. As a result it causes neurological damage. According to the New England Journal of Medicine (Feb 2011) as many as 42% of patients who undergo a bypass are expected to perform significantly poorer on tests on mental ability 5 years later. Other side-effects are personality changes, memory problem and irritability. The other major concern is that the patients face 1% to 2 % chances of dying in the operating room or suffer heart attack during the procedure.

Under the light of the above concerns it had been reported in major newspapers and journals including Business Week (May 28, 2006) that these two procedures (bypass and angioplasty) should have been a part of archives by now but are still proliferating as they contribute towards a major revenue to the hospitals with cardiac department.

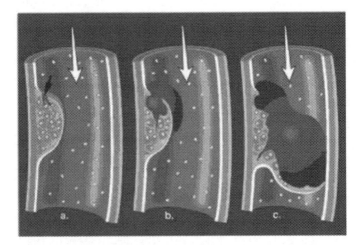

As the plaque is formed, a fibrous cap develops at its top covered by a single layer of endothelium. For a while the protected plaque lies quietly in its place. Eventually the shearing force of blood flowing over the weakened cap may cause it to rupture. The plaque content now oozes out into the flowing bloodstream. To heal the ruptured area, the platelets become activated. They rush to the area and try to stop the invading garbage by clotting the rupture. The clot is self propagating and within minutes the entire artery may become blocked due to clot formation by platelets. With no more blood flowing through the blocked artery, heart muscles may die. This is the definition of heart attack.

More often the doctors equate the plaque accumulated overtime in the artery, like a deposit in the old pipes. As they grow they cause angina (pain) and eventually heart attack. Everyone has had this experience with the household plumbing. First a sink drains slowly and then one day it is so obstructed that it overflows. Many doctors and patients mapped the familiar and intuitive model of pipes into the problem of coronary artery disease.

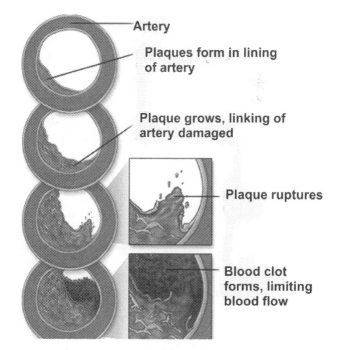

Artery

Plaques form in lining of artery

Plaque grows, linking of artery damaged

Plaque ruptures

Blood clot forms, limiting blood flow

The logic of therapeutic intervention here is clear. Arteries provide the network for blood flow. If the plaque obstruct flow in a patient with chronic angina, then plaque must be removed or the blood must be bypassed. Managing the plaque or unwanted deposits in this way would restore flow, reduce the frequency and severity of angina and prevent damage to the heart muscles. Such plumbing metaphors with all their intuitive appeal, were not simply a way describing and marketing angioplasty and bypass surgery to patients. They also influenced the thinking of the doctors powerfully.

But there is a missing link. One thing that differentiate the plaque deposits in human arteries and the blockage of the house sink is that in 87.5 % of the cases the cause of heart attacks is not the biggest plaque deposits in the arteries ranging from 70 % to 80 % or 90 % blockage but it is the smaller plaque like 30 % or 40% that are responsible for the heart attack as explained previously and managing these smaller plaques through angioplasty and bypass surgery is impossible because these are plenty in numbers.

Since the bypass surgery and angioplasty targets only the biggest plaque this means theoretically by removing the biggest plaque you are reducing the chances of further heart attacks only by 12.5%. But in reality it makes the patient 's condition even more worse.

To understand why angioplasty and bypass surgery cannot improve the life expectancy of patient and rather increases the mortality (death rate). Let's understand how bypass surgery and angioplasty is done.

Look closely at the details of the bypass heart surgery. After an anesthetist renders the patient unconscious, the surgeon removes a portion of artery or veins called graft from the patient's arm or leg or chest. Then rib cage is cut open to stitch the bypass graft to the blocked coronary artery. Angioplasty involves only slightly less bravado. The cardiologist snakes a three foot long balloon tipped catheter into a coronary artery. The balloon ruptures the plaque, stretches the artery wall, and deploys a wire mesh stent to prop it open.

Now the problem with both the procedures is that the body somehow recognizes the surgery sites as dumping site and start pouring deposits and garbage within a few months and the artery again gets blocked.

According to the Archives of Internal Medicine (Medical Journal) Feb 2012, in a randomized trail 7229 patients who had undergone bypass surgery or angioplasty (between 1970 to 2011) were observed and compared with patients with similar severity of blockage but have not gone for surgery. The report concluded that no extra benefits are seen after surgery in patients in comparison to those who avoided surgery. Similar report was published in The New York Times (27 Feb 2012) also. Besides no benefit these surgeries come with many life long side effects. One of them is poor mental ability post surgery. Doctors stop the heart during surgery and the blood is rerouted through the heart lung machine. As a result it causes neurological damage. According to the New England Journal of Medicine (Feb 2011) as many as 42% of patients who undergo a bypass are expected to perform significantly poorer on tests on mental ability 5 years later. Other side-effects are personality changes, memory problem and irritability. The other major concern is that the patients face 1% to 2 % chances of dying in the operating room or suffer heart attack during the procedure.

Under the light of the above concerns it had been reported in major newspapers and journals including Business Week (May 28, 2006) that these two procedures (bypass and angioplasty) should have been a part of archives by now but are still proliferating as they contribute towards a major revenue to the hospitals with cardiac department.

Chapter 5

Road to Heart Disease Goes Through Diabetes, High B.P, High Cholesterol And Obesity

Let's take an imaginary situation where a healthy individual wants to achieve a status of heart disease patient (in 1950's suffering from heart attack was almost a status symbol majorly known to occur to rich and wealthy people). For that many health conditions will take him there namely diabetes, high cholesterol, high B.P and obesity. Now what criteria does he have to fulfill to be a diabetic patient or a patient with high B.P or high cholesterol?

Again it depends on the year to which this imaginary situation belongs. For instance had it been before 1997, a person would have been labelled as diabetic only if his fasting blood sugar threshold was above 140mg/dL but in 1997 the threshold was reduced to 126mg/dL. That means people with fasting blood sugar between 126mg/dL and 140mg/dL who were until now considered to be normal till 1997 became diabetic overnight. Approximately 14% new people joined the existing mass of diabetic patients, which was a great business for the drug companies manufacturing diabetes drugs. No surprise the head of diabetes standard cut off panel were the paid consultants to Aventis Pharmaceuticals, Bristol-Myers Squibb, Eli Lilly and Company, GlaxoSmithKline, Novartis, Merck and Pfizer—all of which make diabetes drugs.

Similar was the case of hypertension till 1997. Individuals having more than 160mmhg systolic B.P and 100mmhg diastolic B.P were considered as hypertension patients. However the standard was dropped in 1997 to 140mmhg systolic B.P and 90mmhg diastolic B.P. This means an additional 35% new population became high B.P patients overnight. Again 9 out of 11 panelists for setting standards of high blood pressure guidelines had some kind of financial ties either as paid consultants, paid speakers or grant recipients to the drug companies that made B.P lowering drugs.

When more people are categorized as patients the only people who gain are pharmaceutical companies as is evident from the American Court Verdict on 2nd July 2012 where Glaxosmithkline was held guilty of conspiring, educating and bribing doctors for profit and promoting medicines for uses for which they were not licensed. Glaxosmithkline was fined 3 billion dollars for this misconduct and was also convicted in July 2013 by the Chinese govt. for similar fraud.

Similarly till 1998, cholesterol level of more than 240mg/dL was considered to be fit for an individual to go for lowering cholesterol through drug therapy. However in 1998 the cholesterol level standard was lowered to 200mg/dL. That means a massive 86 % new population joined the existing mass of high cholesterol patients. Here also eight of the nine experts who lowered the standard cholesterol level were paid consultant to drug companies making cholesterol lowering drugs.

Although in the above cases the profit motive is clearly visible but there is one more dimension to the setting of standards for diabetes, high B.P, high cholesterol or other such health conditions which indicates that blindly following these health parameters itself can be unhealthy for you. In most of the cases the standard were set keeping in mind the Americans which can hardly be standardized for the rest of the world. For example let's take a case reported in "The China Study". It was discovered that blood cholesterol level for rural Chinese adults averaged 127 mg/dL, with individual village averages ranging 88-165 mg/dL. At that time (mid-1980s), 127 mg/dL was considered dangerously low. The "normal" range for serum cholesterol in the United States at that time was 155-274 mg/dL (with an average of 212 mg/dL), and there was some surprising evidence among Western subjects that incidences of suicides, accidents, and violence as well as colon cancer were higher when total cholesterol levels were below 160 mg/dL. Should it therefore be assumed that virtually all rural Chinese were on a high risk range for suicides, accidents, violence, and colon cancer!

Of course, they found nothing of the sort. Instead, they discovered that the Chinese villagers averaging 127 mg/dL were actually far healthier than Americans with so-called normal cholesterol levels. Dr T. Colin first thought was that perhaps their cholesterol assay method (how they collected and analyzed the blood samples) might be faulty. Following Popper's principle of trying to disprove his own hypothesis.

He tried to discredit his own finding by using another assay method and repeating these analyses at laboratories in three different locations (Cornell, Beijing and London). All the analyses showed the same low cholesterol levels. Now they had to make sense of the apparent paradox that the healthiest Chinese people had cholesterol levels that would have been considered dangerously low in the United States. Further examination revealed that for this Chinese range of 88-165 mg/dL like the U.S. range of 155-274 mg/dL lower levels of cholesterol were associated with increased protection from several cancers and related serious diseases. The Chinese population showed correlations between low cholesterol and health that could not be observed in the United States because almost no Americans had cholesterol that low. The Chinese range showed that cholesterol of 88 mg/dL could be healthier than cholesterol of 155 mg/dL a finding that simply could not have been extracted from a study of U.S. population.

The point is whatever is standardized in one part of the world cannot be adopted elsewhere. Then there are other factors like White Coat Syndrome or White Coat Hypertension. It is the moment when the patient is in the doctor's chamber and his, blood pressure hikes at the sight of the doctor. More the doctor commands respect more would be the shift of blood pressure from his natural blood pressure. This means the blood pressure measured at this moment is not the correct one but the temporarily raised one and it happens as many as in 70% of the cases. This means the reading of blood pressure taken for prescribing the medicine can be misleading and far from the actual dose of medicine needed by the patient.

And finally how the drug will work for the patient may vary from individual to individual depending upon many factors including genes, race, continent and the metabolic rate of the individual at the time of taking the drug.

Above it there is a great deal of variation in the understanding of the expectation of performance of a particular drug as is evident from a trial called ALLHAT (short for Antihypertensive and Lipid-Lowering Treatment to Prevent Heart Attack Trial). This was a mammoth trial of the treatment of high blood pressure (hypertension). Although it received some support from Pfizer, it was mainly supported and organized by the National Heart Lung and Blood Institute—a part of National Institutes of Health (NIH). The ALLHAT study was eight years long and involved 42,000 people at more than six hundred clinics, the largest clinical trial of the treatment of high blood pressure ever done. It compared four types of drugs: (1) a calcium channel blocker—sold by Pfizer as Norvasc, the fifth best selling drug in the world in 2002; (2) an alpha-adrenergic blocker—sold by Pfizer as Cardura, and also sold generically as doxazosin; (3) an angiotensin-converting-enzyme (ACE) inhibitor—sold by AstraZeneca as Zestril and by Merck as Prinivil, and also sold generically as Lisinopril and (4) a generic diuretic ("Water pill") of a type that has been on the market for over fifty years.

The results, reported in 2002 in The Journal of the American Medical Association, were startling. To nearly everyone's surprise, the old time diuretic turned out to be just as good for lowering blood pressure, and actually better for preventing some of the devastating complications of high blood pressure—mainly heart disease and strokes.

Participants treated with the diuretic were much less likely to develop heart failure than those treated with Norvasc. And they were less likely to develop heart failure, strokes, and a number of other complications than those treated with the ACE inhibitor. As for Cardura, that part of the trial had to be stopped early, because so many people who received that drug developed heart failure. The director of the National Heart Lung, and Blood Institute was unequivocal in his conclusion. "ALLHAT shows that diuretics are the best choice to treat hypertension both medically and economically."

Yet over the years the newer drugs have largely supplanted diuretics as treatment for high blood pressure. Diuretics were not promoted because generic manufacturers don't usually spend money on marketing. In contrast, when the new drugs came to the market they were promoted incessantly.

Now let's assume the standard set for diabetes or high B.P. or high Cholesterol suit an individual's physical make up of the body and he is diagnosed appropriately and given an appropriate dose of a drug which worked favorable as expected. Then comes the side effects. For instance diabetes drug Actos increases the risk of bladder cancer by 40%. Banned in many countries including France and Germany in September 2010, in India it is sold as Pioglitazone/Pioglar and Poiz among others. Although briefly banned in India in 2013, the ban was lifted following protest by certain groups of pharmaceutical companies and lobbying of certain group of physicians. More over by the time serious side effects of the present drugs is established it would have already killed lakhs of patients. The broadminded doctors are over enthusiastic about the newly released drugs impatiently waiting to see its effects/consequences in patients. For example new drugs like Sitagliptin, all target GLP-1 a peptide that is released in the gut when you eat. GLP-1 normally acts to trigger the release of insulin from the beta cells in the pancreas so by manipulating its level, these drugs are a more sophisticated version of the old Glutamine drugs which also stimulate the beta cells to produce insulin.

Glutamine produce the same boost to insulin release regardless of how much you have eaten. However new drugs are sensitive to your meal size. This means that the amount of GLP-1 produced and the amount of insulin released is appropriate to your food intake. As you know making more insulin isn't such a good idea because excess insulin itself is harmful.

In general the new drugs increase the amount of GLP-1 that's produced at meal times to compensate for the loss of insulin sensitivity and overcome the decline in production that often occurs in people with diabetes. One approach is to make the GLP-1 produced stay active for longer by blocking an enzymes called DPP-4 whose job in turn is to clear away GLP-1.

But here the serious concern is more serious because the job of the blocked enzymes DPP-4 isn't just to clear away GLP-1, it cleans up a number of other bodily processes that you don't want to go on for too long (Such as inflammation) and targets cells that are turning cancerous. There have been some early reports of raised risk of inflammatory problems in patients with rheumatoid arthritis and of cancer particularly melanoma, prostrate and lung.

The side effects involving cholesterol lowering drugs, diabetes drugs and drugs for B.P. are quite substantial as they don't work the way it is illusioned by the general mass and sometime even by the doctor. Let's take the case of cholesterol lowering drug "(Statin)". It does not directly lower the Cholesterol. It works by inhibiting an enzyme that is crucial to the manufacture of cholesterol by the body (An enzyme is a specialized protein that helps to speed up a chemical reaction. For example, our digestive enzymes help speed up the breakdown of food into simple chemicals that can then be absorbed into the body). Statin also increases the uptake of LDL cholesterol by the liver, another way in which they lower the blood level of cholesterol. The enzyme that is inhibited by statin work very early on in the synthetic pathway (the synthetic pathway is like the assembly line in a factory; it is set of chemical processes that occur in side cells as the body manufacturers molecules it needs to survive). When this enzyme is inhibited the levels of other important molecules, such as coenzyme Q10 (learn more about that later), can also drop in people taking these medications.

Conclusively we can say that right from diagnosis of diabetes, high B.P. and high cholesterol to choosing the right drug in right doses is a total hit and trial method of expecting a cure often dangerously damaging for the patients.

As it is clear from the 2011 Cochrane Report (Supreme Authority among Reports and Journals). The Cochrane authors reviewed data from 14 trials involving 34,272 patients. Outcomes in patients given statins were compared with outcomes in patients given placebo or usual care. Result suggested that there is not enough evidence to recommend the widespread use of statins in the primary prevention of heart disease.

Why the cholesterol lowering drug may not help in the prevention of heart diseases can be made clear through the Harvard Research Publication-2012, where researchers have discovered that LDL can be distinguished in two categories based on the size i.e. small LDL and large LDL. Of them the small LDL is damaging, because of their small size they penetrate into the endothelial wall of the arteries resulting in inflammation and arterial blockage.

This means two patients with the same raised high LDL may not have the same risk of heart disease but to find which of the patient is having the raised small sized LDL, one has to go through a very specialized High Tech Nuclear Magnetic Resonance Imaging Technology which is till now not available in India and may cost you around $ 200 per test elsewhere in the world.

So now it is even more understandable that once a patient takes the route of drug therapy for the treatment of diabetes or high B.P. or high cholesterol he can never be off medicine. He has to be continuously on an ever increasing dose of drugs lifelong more often leading to further complication like heart disease, cancer etc.

To free yourself from the clutches of lifelong medicine and to return back to your healthy state you must take the route of "The China Study" Diet Plan as explained in chapter 6. No matter how severe may be your health condition at this moment or you may be on drugs for many years, still you can bounce back with the China Study Diet Plan and remain healthy & drug free lifelong.

The Obesity Mafia

I had to include this section in the book as you know that an obese person has 100% chances of suffering from heart disease as obesity burdens the heart to a great extent.

To understand how obesity leads to heart failure let's assume that your heart is like a Maruti 800 car engine but is wrongly fitted to the body of the truck. How far do you think the tiny engine (heart) will be able to carry the oversized truck (your body)? Obese people remain obese in spite of their all efforts to reduce weight because they put their effort in wrong direction and the credit for misunderstanding of the solution to reduce weight goes to slimming centres like the VLCC and fitness centers etc. Behavior of these slimming centers reminds me of a Leaking Tap Analogy. Let's say you complain of leakage of a tap in your bathroom. If I give you the solution by stopping the supply of water to your house and hence leakage in the tap also stops. That's exactly how these slimming centers work. They put customers on fat/calorie less diet As a result the customer reduces weight temporarily but after some time returns back to the centre again with same complain. It may be profitable for slimming centers' but damaging for patients desperate to lose weight. Understand the simple science and you can never be obese.

Excess calorie # excess body weight
Excess acid food= excess body weight

This means to lose weight you have to eat more and more alkaline diet. The diet which once eaten turns into acidic waste must be avoided. This means if you give up refined (oil, salt sugar), processed/packed food and milk products and if you can live more and more on fruits and raw vegetables you may lose weight @ 10% of the body weight per month till you achieve your optimum weight. This is the fastest and most healthiest way of reducing weight permanently.

Endnote: Now you have understood that trying to treat one of the health conditions (high cholesterol, high B.P, diabetes, obesity and heart failure) may lead to other diseases as the above five health conditions are closely related. So by the mid of the this year the clever pharmaceutical giants are ready to launch all cure pills called polypills. Here they are combining all the drugs together i.e statin + metformin + asprin + ACE – inhibitor = polypil with the hope that it will make a good marketing sense (according to Journal of American Medical Association). But try to understand (as I explained in the chapter Jiyo Jee Bhar Ke) that once a nutrient or a compound enters the body, the way it will react inside the body totally depends on whether it has entered in isolation or in combination with other compounds/drugs. In this case the way metformin may work in the body when taken alone may not be the same or may be even opposite when it is combined with other compounds or drugs. In case of polypills it is not just the case of 2 drugs combination; here it is 4. This means the variety of ways in which it may react in the body of the patients is in geometric progression and estimating the side effects accurately is possible and understandable only when it is tried on thousands of patients and all those patients are being followed for at least 10 yrs. This is the only scientific way available to medical science as of now which you trust but that means if you are the one who is given a new drug means you are one of the guinea pigs for that particular drug.

Chapter 6

No One Can Die of
A Heart Disease

I can tell you two things about this chapter.

One: The story you are going to read has the potential to make all the cardiologists jobless.

Two: After reading this chapter you will never need to make any further visit to the doctor for the treatment of diabetes, high cholesterol, high B.P, obesity or heart disease.

I believe that this is the most powerful story in the history of medical science, but kept out of the medical college syllabus as it can make the entire hospital system obsolete and useless.

Till the beginning of 18 century two of the world's healthiest civilizations called Hunza and Pima Indians were living near Kashmir (India). They were known to live beyond 100 years of their age and were majorly disease free throughout their life. Their longevity was mostly attributed to their lifestyle and food habits. It was at this time the Pima Indian's decided to migrate to Arizona near America. Pima Indians got settled in Arizona and continued with the same lifestyle of majorly agriculture business and same food style, as it was when they were with Hunza. They remained healthy and disease free till 1960's. In 1960's American Govt. offered the Pima Indians to trade their occupied land to American Govt. and against that American Govt. promised them to give lifelong supply of food. As agreed the Pima Indians started getting the supply of packed/fast food. By 1970 Pima Indians were recognized worldwide for their achievement of being now known to be the world's sickest civilization with all the members of the community suffering single or multiple medical conditions such as heart diseases, diabetes, high cholesterol, high B.P, obesity and other life style diseases. They became the centre of attraction for major pharmaceutical companies as they could get human guinea pigs for their experimental drugs at a very cheap price and in abundance with multiple combinations and degree of diseases. It was the time around 1970 to 1975, some researchers handpicked and gathered some of the members of Pima Indians with various ailments namely heart disease, diabetes, high cholesterol, high B.P and obesity and decided to put the targeted Pima Indians in their original diet which they used to consume as is still consumed by Hunza Indians.

To the surprise of researchers within 1 to 1 1/2 years their disease pattern reversed. The blood pressure and cholesterol level significantly reduced. Blood glucose fell in normal range, weight reduced appreciably and clogged arteries cleared up. It was clear that the food which can help in preventing a disease can also help in reversing a disease.

Now the question is what's the magic recipe which helped Hunza Civilization to live disease free and helped Pima Indians to reverse their disease status. My mentor Dr. T. Colin Campbell approximately put it as The China Study Diet Plan. Dr Caldwell Esselsytyn in one of his lectures described it as followed.

WHAT NOT TO EAT:

- You may not eat anything that has a mother or a face (no meat, poultry or fish)
- You cannot eat dairy products.
- You must not consume oil of any kind—not even a drop.
- No sugar, salt and refined products.

WHAT TO EAT

- All vegetables (in unprocessed form, in their natural state).
- All legumes (beans, peas and lentils of all varieties)
- All whole grains (in unrefined state)
- All seasonal Fruits

Above is what resembles closely to the diet of Hunza civilization that researches attribute their longevity to the very specific diet. There are six more civilizations in the modern world where there is no trace of heart disease. These are Okinawa of Japan, Bama of China, Vilicabamba of Equador, Abhkasia of Goergia, Compodimele of Italy and Symi of Greece.

Besides being known for their longevity, they have one more thing in common that is their diet which is similar to the above diet as suggested by Dr. Caldwell Esselsytyn.

The connection between Whole Food Plant Based Diet and reversal of lifestyle disease was established many times. One of the well-known was the example of World War-II. During that period the heart attacks and diabetes fell by 50% in England. It was established that during the world war sugar consumption fell because of shipping hazards in high sea. No sifting of whole wheat flour into refined flour could take place because of scarcity of energy. The govt. encouraged people to plant victory gardens to source their food. The people were forced to consume diet which was resembled closely with The China Study Diet. This resulted in unexpected fall in heart attacks and diabetes rate by almost 50%. But soon after the war was over, the citizens got back to their original refined and processed diet the rate of heart attack and diabetes returned to the previous height.

Similar evidence could be established from the story of Eskimos of Northern Yakon territory (Canada) who were known for their robust health till 1955 when they were primarily nomad food gatherer. The Canadian Govt. offered them jobs in Defence Early Warning System (DEW). As a result they were forced to eat 100% modern refined, processed and packed food shipped from outside. Within a decade women suffered from gall bladder attacks and diabetes and men developed coronary artery disease. A team of doctors from Alberta changed their diet to raw and whole plant based food. As a result within 2 years the disease pattern reversed. Since late 19th century many doctors around the world have indicated and established and practiced the science of human body (as I hinted in Chapter1) that you can reverse your disease just by changing your diet pattern. Even today many modern doctors (refer chapter 7) practice and heal people just with the power of 'The China Study Diet Plan'.

How healthy is the China Study Diet Plan?

To make it understandable Dr. T. Colin Campbell, the chief scientist of 'The China Study' (biggest ever study on Human Nutrition) puts it beautifully as under:

"Let's pretend that all its effects could be achieved through a drug. Imagine a big pharmaceutical company holding a press conference to unveil a new pill called Eunutria. They unveil a list of scientifically proven effects of Eunutria that includes the following,

- Prevents 95 percent of all cancers, including those caused by environmental toxins.
- Prevents nearly all heart attacks and strokes.
- Reverses even severe heart disease.
- Prevents and reverses type 2 diabetes so quickly and effectively that after three days on drug, it's dangerous for users to continue to use insulin.
- What about side effects, you ask? Of course there are side effects. They include:
- Gets you to your ideal weight in a healthy and sustainable fashion.
- Eliminates most migraines, acne, colds and flu, chronic pain and intestinal distress.
- Improves energy

- Cures erectile dysfunction (that makes the pill a blockbuster success all by itself.
- Those are just the side effects for individuals taking the pill.
- There are also environmental effects,
- Slows and possibly reverses global warming
- Reduces groundwater contamination
- Ends the need for deforestation
- Shuts down factory farms
- Reduces malnutrition and dislocation among the world's poorest citizens.

How healthy is 'The China Study Diet Plan'? It is hard to imagine anything healthier—or anything more effective at addressing our biggest health issues. Not only is The China Study Diet Plan the healthiest way of eating that has ever been studied, but it's far more effective in promoting health and preventing disease than prescription drugs, surgery, vitamin and herbal supplementation and genetic manipulation.

If 'The China Study Diet Plan' were a pill, its inventor would be the wealthiest person on earth. Since it is not a pill, no market forces conspire to advocate for it. No mass media campaign promotes it. No insurance coverage pays for it. Since it is not a pill and nobody has figured out how to get hugely wealthy by showing people how to eat it, the truth has been buried by half-truths, unverified claims and downright lies. The concerted effort of many powerful interests to ignore, discredit, and hide the truth has worked so far."

Now if we compare how 'The China Study diet' performs when we compare it against modern medicines and surgical interventions we must compare across the following three parameters,

- How quickly does it work? (Rapidity)
- How many health problems does it help solve?(Breadth)
- How much will my health improves due to the intervention?(Depth)

Let 's look at each of these in turn.

Rapidity

How long does it take for a nutrient drug, genetic modification or whatever to actually function within the body? I am not talking about how long it takes for a substance to be absorbed in the blood stream and transported to the tissue cells. Instead I am asking, "How long before there's a meaningful effect, like an energy boost or reduction of disease symptoms!"

The speed at which most nutritional benefits appear when switching to a 'The China Study diet' is jaw-dropping. Diabetics must be monitored from the very first day they adopt the diet, so their medicines can be reduced as the diet takes effects. Otherwise they are in real danger of having their blood sugar drop low enough to send them into hypoglycemic shock.

Non nutritious food also works really quickly, but in the opposite direction. Within one to four hours of consuming, for example a high-fat Mc-Donald's meal (Egg McMuffin,

Sausage Mcmuffin, two hash brown patties, non caffeinated beverages) serum triglycerides shoot up (increasing the risk of heart disease and diabetes as well as many other conditions) and arteries stiffen (raising blood pressure). Recovery to normal fluidity takes several hours. None of this occurs following a low fat meal consisting of cereal and fruits.

Another professor of Campbell University, Dr. Caldwell Esselstyn, Jr MD used 'The China Study Diet Plan' to reverse advanced heart disease in a study that began in 1985. He found that chronic chest pain (also known as angina) typically disappeared within one to two weeks. Compare that to an angina drug such as Ranolazine (marketed under the trade name Ranexa) which was approved by the Food and Drug Administration (FDA) in 2006. One clinical trial undertaken to establish its effectiveness randomly assigned 565 patients to a Ranexa group or a placebo group. The Ranexa group experienced a "Statistically significant reduction in angina episodes over six weeks". Sounds great right? What it means is that the Ranexa Group went from 4.5 to 3.5 angina episodes per week. Not exactly the speedy solution anyone really wants, is it? Add to it the common side effects reported by the manufacturer, including "dizziness, headache, constipation and nausea (the study didn't' say how rapidly those showed up) and you have western medicine's best answer to a 'The China Study Diet Plan'; expensive interventions with limited positive effect and a host of potential side effects.

Some may think it's unfair to compare pharmaceuticals to 'The China Study Diet Plan', since the drugs are meant to treat symptoms rather than root cause of a disease. But if there is one thing these prescription meds should have going for them, it is rapidity of effect. Indeed the one useful function they can perform is "buying time" for patients for whom a lifestyle and dietary intervention otherwise might be too late. When someone is wheeled into the ER after suffering a heart attack or stroke, it's a better idea to administer a thrombolytic drug to dissolve the blood clot than to give them an intravenous spinach smoothie, but aside from true emergencies, the rapidity of response of 'The China Study Diet Plan' is superior to any drug—without the negative side effect.

Breadth

Let's imagine that some blind men assumed responsibility for an elephant's health and well-being. What would this look like? Obviously, none of the blind men would be tasked with monitoring the whole elephant—that would be impossible! Each would focus on his own area of "expertise": the leg, the tusk, the trunk, the tail, the ear, and the belly. If the elephant ate some moldy peanuts and began developing liver cancer, none of the blind men would notice, as none of the parts they were tasked with monitoring would be sufficiently affected yet. Only when the cancer reached a critical mass would its symptoms become noticeable: first as decreased appetite that the "trunk doctor" would notice, next as intestinal distress that the "tail doctor" would certainly smell, and ultimately as a fever that the "ear doctor" could sense and measure. The blind men, limited by their experience of the elephant as a collection of individual, unrelated parts, have no ability to discern and deal with root causes that precede symptoms. By necessity, their treatments will react to problems that have already developed rather than preventing those problems in the first place. This is also the first major characteristic of our disease-care system: reactivity, because the blind men can discern symptoms but not causes, they treat those symptoms as if they were the entire problem. The trunk doctor might sugar-coat the moldy peanuts in an attempt to stimulate the elephant's appetite. The tail doctor, having no way to intervene in the elephant's gastrointestinal workings, might just fit the poor creature with a large carbon-filter diaper and explain that modern medicine doesn't really have a cure for that sort of thing. And the ear doctor might treat the ear fever with ice packs and declare the elephant "cured" once the ear temperature returned to normal. This is also the case with our disease-care system: it focuses on treating symptoms as if they were root causes and as a result, it tends to choose interventions that completely ignore the true root causes and thus make it highly likely that symptoms will reappear.

That is how the treatment happens in today arena of Super Specialty Hospitals, where it is being educated and believed that for one disease there should be one medicine, they never heal the body in totality. Whereas you will know in detail in this chapter that single most important reason of the life style diseases such as diabetes, heart disease, high cholesterol, high B.P., is the ill health of the blood vessel i.e. Vascular System of the Body. 'The China Study Diet Plan' works towards healing the vascular network of the body thus working simultaneously across all the diseases rather than working toward one disease at a time.

Depth

It is commonly heard from the doctor that once you are diagnosed with diabetes or for that matter high B.P. etc. you may be able to control it with drugs but you have to live with this disease.

You will never be able to cure yourself of the disease. Bypass patients going for repeated bypass or angioplasty patient developing blockage at the same location within 6 months of the surgery are very common. It is clear that the allopathic method of treatment work on the superficial level and their approach is never to cure the patient for the root cause. Whereas from my own experience through the patients who visit my clinic or the one who joined my health workshops, can tell you that 'The China Study Diet Plan' addresses the cause of the disease and within a span of 3 to 6 months the patient following The China Study Diet Plan is totally cured of the disease and rarely had to go back to take the same allopathic route.

Now the bigger question could be how 'The China Study Diet Plan' can help reverse a disease? You may be interested in exploring the science behind it. Consider the following explanation. Our body consists of a vast network of blood vessels long enough to stretch from the earth to the moon. Your health primarily depends on the health of your blood vessels and the health of blood vessels is majorly controlled and reflected by the health of the innermost layer of the blood vessel known as endothelium. When we talk of coronary artery diseases it is mostly the plaque deposits on endothelium (inner layer). In case of high cholesterol the endothelial layer becomes sticky and attracts cholesterol and fatty substances to stick to it. In case of high blood pressure the endothelial layer becomes stiff resulting in the rise of blood pressure. In case of diabetes the endothelial layer near the pancreatic region becomes inflamed triggering various reactions including the condition of insulin resistance. If you protect your endothelial layers of "blood vessels" from inflammation, plague deposit and stiffening, you can protect yourself from majority a of lifestyle diseases including heart disease, diabetes, high cholesterol and high B.P. Maintaining a good endothelial layer health can help you maintain optimum body weight and shed excess fat. Now the next question is how to maintain a good endothelial layer health? To explain this I will take the help of 1998 Noble Prize Winning Science of Dr. Louis J. Ignarro. To maintain good health the endothelial layer of the blood vessels produce Nitric Oxide (NO) which is absolutely essential to maintain one's health,

Find below the function of NO (Nitric Oxide) in our body.

1) 'It relaxes blood vessels, selectively boosting blood flow to the organ that needs it. Therefore regulates the blood pressure and keeps it to the optimum level.

2) It prevents white blood cells and platelets from becoming sticky, and thus stopping the building of plaque deposits and stopping the progress of heart attacks.

3) It keeps the smooth muscles cells of arteries from developing plaque also resulting in keeping the cholesterol level to optimum.

4) It helps heal inflammation at various locations in the inner lining (endothelial) of the blood vessels including the inner lining of the blood vessels in pancreatic region resulting in proper functioning of insulin, thus reversing diabetes.

5) It increases the metabolic rate of the body resulting in burning of the excess fat thus helping to shed excess body weight.

For the above reason Nitric Oxide is sometimes known as a Miracle Molecule.

To understand how plant based nutrition facilitates nitric oxide production, you need to have a sense of the biochemistry. The essential building block for nitric oxide production is a substance called L-arginine, an amino acid that is in rich supply in a variety of plant food, especially legumes beans, soy, and nuts. L-arginine which is an amino acid fits neatly into the enzymatic action of nitric oxide of synthase, which then produces nitric oxide from the arginine and oxygen. However, as you can also see in the figure given below, there is a competitor for nitric acid synthase: asymmetric dimethyl arginine or, ADMA, which is manufactured by our bodies in the course of normal protein metabolism. When we have too much ADMA, then L-arginine is edged out for a position in nitric oxide synthase, and the production of nitric oxide fails. There is another delicate enzyme with a formidable name—dimethyl arginine dimethyl amino hydrolase, or DDHA—that destroys ADMA, in order to favor production of nitric oxide. But the usual cardiovascular risk factors (high cholesterol, high triglycerides, high homocysteine, insulin resistance, hypertension and tobacco use) all impair the ability of that delicate enzyme to destroy ADMA.

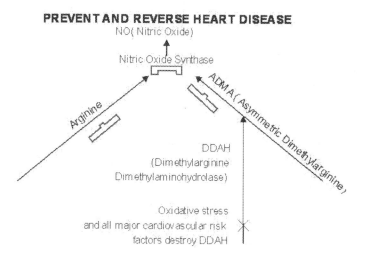

PREVENT AND REVERSE HEART DISEASE

NO(Nitric Oxide)

Nitric Oxide Synthase

ADMA (Asymmetric Dimethylarginine)

Arginine

DDAH
(Dimethylarginine
Dimethylaminohydrolase)

Oxidative stress
and all major cardiovascular risk
factors destroy DDAH

Showing the pathway of nitric oxide production—Arginine through nitric oxide—can be can be blocked by too much ADMA.

This biochemistry explains what is perhaps the key mechanism through which my patients become heart-attack-proof beyond twenty years. Their plant-based diet reduced or entirely eliminated all the above cardiovascular risk factors. The more the patient complied to it, the more he or she reduced the risks. Along the way, they also reduced symptoms such as a angina pectoris-chest pain, perhaps the most frightening and incapacitating symptom of heart disease. Normally, physical efforts or strong emotion causes the endothelium to go into action, producing nitric oxide, dilating the blood vessels, and thus boosting the flow of blood to the heart muscle, but in a patient with coronary disease, endothelium's capacity is badly diminished. His narrowed coronary arteries do not dilate, and therefore his heart muscle does not receive the flow of blood it needs. The result: pain. It may be mild or it may be excruciating. Many patients become 'cardiac cripples', terrified of exerting themselves physically, of making love, of expressing or experiencing strong emotions. To give such patients lasting relief, it is essential to bring more blood to the heart muscles—despite the fact that the blood must flow through partially blocked coronary arteries. How! By restoring endothelium' capacity to manufacture more nitric oxide. The effects of radical shift in nutrition are breathtaking, dramatic and swift.

Those who maintain their food consumption limited to plants and in whole form (not refined, processed and packed) maintain a good blockage free inner layer of the blood vessels. We got the evidence of it during my visit to the longest military tunnel in Vietnam (made during Vietnam War). The document of the autopsy reports of soldiers during the Vietnam war showed the effect of America's artery clogging diet even on very young American Soldiers. The arteries of Vietnamese soldiers were largely clean and free of fatty deposits. Almost 80% of American Battlefield Consolation reports showed gross evidence of coronary artery diseases— clogging and damage that had the soldiers lived, would have grown worse with every passing decade. On the other hand the clean deposit free arteries of Vietnam declared soldiers can clearly be linked to their traditional diet pattern which is largely free of refined, processed and packed food and more of raw or steamed plant based nutrition occupying as much as 80 % of their total diet. I got several occasions to dine with the Buddhist monks of Vietnam and could easily relate that their disease free life can be associated with their diet which closely resembles 'The China Study Diet Plan' and it explains why 3/4th of the planet never suffers from heart disease. It's the industrial nation which is obsessed by the refined, processed and packed food leading to the number one killer zAt this point it is important to remind you that through angiography, the cardiologist aims at detecting the major blockage i.e 70% to 80 % or 90 % and through angioplasty/stenting and bypass surgery, they try to eliminate the larger blockages whereas for 90 % of the heart attacks it is not the larger i.e 70 % and beyond blockages that are responsible rather it is the 30 % to 40 % blockages that may actually be more likely to cause heart attack.

Why? Since there is a significant amount of plaque in your arteries, it's more likely to be calcified and stable. Also, over time, new blood vessels called collaterals grow around blocked arteries—a type of 'built-in bypass'. So if an artery becomes completely obstructed, a heart attack may not necessarily ensue since there is another pathway for blood to flow around the blockage.

In contrast, an artery that is only 30 to 40 percent clogged has not had time to grow new collateral vessels. Also, it is not likely to be calcified and stable, so there is a greater risk of it constricting during times of emotional stress. When an artery in your heart constricts, it may cause rupture in plaques that are weakened, called vulnerable plaques.

When a plaque ruptures, an artery may go from 30 to 40 percent clogged to 100 percent clogged within seconds. This is called "catastrophic progression" (it's as bad as it sounds) and may lead to a heart attack, stroke, or sudden cardiac death. Plaque rupture can occur due to sudden physical or emotional stress.

This explains why the studies I mentioned in chapter 4 failed to show that angioplasty or bypass surgery prolongs life or prevents heart attack in most patients. Most doctors are not going to put stents or a bypass graft in an artery that's only 30 percent blocked because they are often in plenty and technically it is not possible to address each one of them through angioplasty or bypass surgery, yet these are the ones that are most likely to cause a heart attack.

Whereas by putting yourself on 'The China Study Diet Plan' you give your body an opportunity to produce Nitric Oxide, which results in clearing all the blockage including 30% 40% to 90% and 100% blockage. Along with that Nirtic Oxide initiates and accelerates once more the amazing mechanism of the body. It's called arteriogenesis. It is the body's own ability to construct new arteries specially the path when some of the arteries are nearly blocked to reroute the blood through a different path. It is also known as body's own natural bypass by the medical community. This mechanism of the body is not just limited to heart, it is extended to all the organs. It also explains how Nitric Oxide cures the erectile dysfunction among the males which is the basis of how the Viagra works towards penile erection. But beware as I explained in chapter 3 that you attempt to compensate the body's nutritional requirement through the supplement/pills may sabotage and hijack the whole biochemistry of the body. For body's ability to produce Nitric Oxide you must follow 'The China Study Diet Plan'. You must not resort to artificial medium such as steroids to enhance body's ability to produce Nitric Oxide as is often practiced nowadays by most of the body builders and some of the actors.

In London 2012 Olympics you might hae seen some weight lifters inhaling something very strongly, a few seconds before the final lift. Well this is Nitric Oxide—and this is real chemical cheating. They can't be caught as the effect wears away before the lab test.

Actors like Hritik Roshan, Shahrukh Khan, Amir Khan and more recently Farhan Akhtar suddenly pop up within a month with great muscles and six packs due to Nitric Oxide steriod supplements specially made for athletes and body builders. These chemicals are bad for health but Nitric oxide produced by the body's chemical factory is natural, healthy and without side effects.

You may ask how can I claim that the sudden robust, muscular body is the result of consuming steroids and not the result of healthy food and hard long workout.

To understand it, take the analogy of Dr. Verma of Safdarjung Hospital (as elaborated in chapter 7). He was caught by income tax department for having assets near to 10 crores whereas his salary is approximately Rs 70,000/- per month. This means to accumulate Rs 10 crore he has to work for 119 years of his life. Assuming he saved 100% of the salary during that period, which is impossible. His inability to explain the gap between income and the accumulation of wealth amount to a fraud resulting in his landing into jail. Similarly in the history of human beings it is impossible to develop that kind of six packs in a matter of months or so.

It is biologically disputable, otherwise can anyone explain that lakhs of youngsters who go for serious gyming for 3 years can never match the physique of handful of actors who in a matter of time can achieve six packs. and within no time shed the muscles with the excuse that their next movie demands muscleless character. No surprise these actors had to make equal numbers of foreign visits for solving the medical complications they face as a result of it and the number of visits abroad they make for their shooting. So the final words are—stick to 'The China Study Diet Plan' as give your body a chance to heal and reverse the disease you are suffering from. This is what I recommended to the patients visiting my clinic as well as to the participants attending my health workshops. When I argue the same with the learned doctors; why they never educate and give their patients the option of taking the route of healthy healing through the modification of diet, they more often answer saying people may not stick to the 'The China Study Diet Plan' and that it is easier for patients to pop some pills lifelong even if it may not mean cure and may complicate the body's system further. Whereas the truth is when I interact with my patients they say, "doctor please advise me anything you may like so that I do not have to go under the knife". After all who would like to sign an agreement giving consent to the surgeon that if he dies during the surgery, it is entirely his risk knowing that there is a fair chance of the worse happening as the doctors are always referred as practicing doctor or practicing surgeon and till the last day of their retirement doctor's keep on practicing at the cost of patient's health and wealth. With My experience I can tell you that it is always easier to follow a healthy 'The China Study Diet Plan' than popping pills lifelong. That is the reason why it is clear from the report published in the journal of American Medical Association that two third of the patients who are prescribed statin drugs quit taking them just 12 months later.

Chapter 7

Ab Tak Chappan—
The Obsession for Numbers

It was a usual day for me, one of my health workshops was going on, in some part of the world. This time it was in Kuwait Medical Association Auditorium. Everything was going on as usual till I started presenting the successful case histories of the patients whom I cured with 'The China Study Diet Plan' and lifestyle modification (who were otherwise strongly recommended for bypass surgery/angioplasty). One of the participants (most probably a cardiac surgeon) raised an objection pointing out and saying, "you are not a doctor, then how can you treat a patient"? Though my answer was spontaneous but this incidence bugged me for the next few days (and also gave me the courage to write this book). I asked the participant, can you tell me the definition of the word "doctor"? He looked at me in disbelief as to why am I asking him such a stupid question? I continued by giving him the reference of the prestigious medical journal—The Lancet—1999 and also of Wikipedia which says originally a doctor means 'a teacher' or 'a scholar' which still is the meaning of doctor. In the later part of the 18th century some of the medical practitioners started addressing each other as "Doctor" as it commanded a lot of respect and by the end of 19th century medical practitioners almost grabbed the monopoly of using the word" Doctor". That way I truly fit into the definition of "Doctor". Besides clinical practice, I teach people through my health workshops, "How to Reverse a Life Style Disease" through the techniques as discussed in the book. Frankly speaking "You don't need medication, you need education". Now the question is what name will you give to the medical practitioner who is always prescribing medicines and is into the race of surgeries. The dedicatedly professional and single mind tracked modern day physician and medical practitioner. It reminds me of Nana Patekar starer "Ab Tak Chappan" movie where in the race of most numbers of shootouts the Mumbai Police encounter specialist started killing the innocents.

These days surgeons are obsessed with numbers or making world records not in curing and healing patients but in performing or conducting surgeries. If you go through the profile of the so called top cardiologists of India (in their websites), nowhere is the mention of, how many patients remain alive after their bypass surgeries or angioplasties after ten years or for even next one year for that matter. In their profile or bio data they would not like to keep something which may point towards their weakness. Let's have a look at the profile of some of the high profile Indian cardiologists.

1) World record for most number of angioplasties:

Dr Ashok Seth has performed more than 50,000 angiograms and 20,000 angioplasties in his career, for which he has received recognition from "Limca Book of Records" and presently working as Chairman Cardiac Sciences—Fortis Escorts Heart Institute, New Delhi.

My Comments: Don't confuse between number of angioplasty and number of successful angioplasty. Successful angioplasty means the patients may not require angioplasty within 5 years of the first angioplasty.

2) World Record for performing Angioplasty on an oldest (104 yrs) person:

The Padma Vibhushan and Dr. B.C Roy National awardee, Dr Purshotam Lal, an eminent cardiologist and chairman of Metro Hospital and Heart Institute, Noida has set the world record by successfully performing angioplasty with stent on a 104 year old patient from Dehradun to save his life.

My Comments: It is known from the report that the patient (Hari Singh) had undergone angioplasty with stent by Dr Purshotam Lal in 2001also. Had the patient been educated of the diet and lifestyle method (as given in this book), he would not have required either of the two (2001and 2013) angioplasties but then Dr. Purshotam Lal would have missed a chance of creating a world record (which he keeps on flaunting through his in-house newsletters and the notice board of Metro Hospitals).

3) From heart attack to angioplasty in straight 16 minutes: a new National Record:

Dr. Sanjay Rajdev, a consultant cardiologist at Seven Hills Hospital has entered the Limca Book of Records for stopping a heart attack and performing an angioplasty in just 16 minutes against the international standard of 90 minutes.

My Comments: Consider the mandatory steps required once a heart attack patient enters the emergency centre of the hospital.

The steps which need to be followed when a patient with heart attack is taken to the hospital,

- Patient taken to ward on a stretcher
- Shifted to the hospital bed
- Changing of Clothes
- Attaching machines for monitoring
- Monitoring Glucose Level
- Insertion of 2 large bore IVs of normal saline
- Application of defibrillating pads to patient's chest
- Clip bilateral groin hairs
- Prepare for transport to operation theatre
- Place portable monitor and oxygen tank on bed
- Take X-rays

Medication that should be available:

1) Nitroglycerine
2) Asprin
3) Lopressor
4) Plavix

Steps for Angiography:

- Painting the groin
- Injection of local anesthesia

- Inserting the introducer tube
- X-rays taken
- Die insertion
- View the blockage on the monitor
- Steps for Angioplasty:
- Accessing coronary artery
- Insertion of guiding catheter
- Insertion of expert catheter
- Removal of clot from the artery
- Insertion of stent on balloon
- Inflate balloon
- Leave the stent
- Deflate the balloon inject nitroglycerine in the vessel
- Closure of the wound

The above are some of the major steps which a cardiologist had to follow right from admitting a heart attack patient to an emergency ward to conduct angioplasty. Deliberately I have ignored some micro steps (which will be equal in numbers) to make it simple for you. Even if we understand that all the arrangements including availability of doctors/nurses are done while the patient was on the way to the hospital even then seeing the volume of steps it would be humanly impossible for a hospital to conduct the procedure right from heart attack to angioplasty in just 16 minutes.

Now even for a layman it is not difficult to understand that completing the above procedure in less than 90 min (international standard) is not only highly life threatening for the patients but also illegal and highly unethical. Just imagine how it would be that you are transporting a patient with heart attack to a hospital and on the way you are told that through this patient, doctors are going to achieve or break a world record, of "from heart attack to angioplasty in less than 10 minutes". Don't take me wrong, I have no doubt that our skilled cardiologist would be able to achieve even that feat as well but I only fear about the life and health of the patient involved.

You will be surprised to know that the cases given above are not the stray cases of some of the obsessed cardiologist but there are many more stalwarts and Padma Bhushan Award recepient cardiologists in race. Let's peep into the (high) profile of some of the most media managed cardiologists.

1) Dr. Naresh Trehan, cardiac surgeon is honored with Padma Bhushan and Padma Shree Awards and presently working as a Chairman & Managing Director, Medanta—The Medicity and has performed more than 50,000 heart surgeries.

My Comments: With due respect to you for the kind of celebrity status you have achieved (which most film stars would envy) my humble question to you (Dr. Naresh Trehan) is that "why can't a cardiologist talk in terms of number of patients who survived without having undergone repeated surgery within next five years of the surgery rather than talking in terms of number of surgeries performed in the life time. It appears that cardiologists are interested in putting most of the patients visiting them under the knife even though there are safer nonsurgical and more powerful and less expensive intervention (as given in the book) available.

I propose Dr. Naresh Trehan to put forward diagnostic documents of his patients on whom angioplasty/bypass surgery has been performed in last 5 years, for scrutiny as such investigation elsewhere in the world (read ahead in this chapter) resulted in the conviction of large number of cardiologist for performing unnecessary angioplasty/bypass surgeries. These surgeries are very tempting for cardio surgeons as these approximately 1 to 2 hours procedures attract a huge revenue (Rs 5 lakh on an average) which makes the cardiac surgeon see every patient fit for these surgeries.

2) Dr. S.S Bansal: Director of Metro Heart Institute, Faridabad and well known heart surgeon not only has the passion of numbers but also likes to be called first in the country. Recently he is proud of and is flaunting being the 1st to introduce minimal invasive angioplasty with small dimensional 4F lumen catheter from Japan irrespective of the fact whether it is clinically, substantially proven to be a better technology or just you are going to be one of his guinea pigs of his new technologies.

My Comment: Always a new technology is either being equated or automatically qualifies as a better technology but in case of medical sciences it is seldom correct.

Consider the case of stents:

Name	Disadvantages	Picture
1.Ballooning Angioplasty: Inflatable balloon inserted into the blocked vessel in the heart to push the plaque against the vessel wall and restore blood flow.	Restenosis occurs after the angioplasty is done	
2. Bare Metal Stent: Metallic mesh tube implanted into the vessel after balloon angioplasty to restore blood flow to the heart and to keep the vessel open over time.	Because of the presence of a foreign object Plaque forms around the stent	
3.Drug Eluting Stents: Metallic mesh tube coated with drugs to prevent re-narrowing of the blood vessel where the stent is placed	Drug limits the formation of new endothelial layer over the new stent to inhibit clot formation. But this endothelialization is important for vascular healing and for prevention of thrombus formation. Lack of healing caused by antiproliferative drugs can make the stent an exposed surface on which a life threatening clot can form.	
4. Bioresorbable Vascular Scaffold-- 2013: Absorb is a drug-eluting mesh implant made of polylactide a material used in dissolving sutures. Absorb restores blood flow to the heart and then dissolves after doing its job, which may allow natural vessel function to resume.	They are thick and made up of plastic material and may get fractured while implanting leading to complications like bleeding and death .	

To understand how a new technology helps doctors to influence their patients, consider the above example of "evolution of stents". A clinical trial on angioplasty published in 1992 studied a group of patients who had the procedure in 1985," says David Jones "But angioplasty has been refined since 1985. So you start another trial in 1992 and publish in 1998, then the cardiologist say,' now we have fancy stents, not old fashioned stents, they used in 1992.' and so on. As long as you continue to innovate in a way that at face value, looks to be an improvement, the believers can always step out under the weight of negative clinical experience by saying that the research necessarily applies to an earlier state of medical technology, doctors like S.S Bansal can always use the above analogy to influence their patients to choose their hospitals in comparison to other hospitals.

"But one of the dirty secret of cardiac care", says David Jones is that, "until the 1970s, heart expert could not agree on what was causing heart attacks, rendering their interventions equal parts gamble and trial by doing".

Cardiologist like Dr S.S Bansal uses this illusion (new technologies = better technologies) to their favor and every now and then come up with some or the other new offering.

No surprise that Dr. S.S Bansal enjoys nearly a celebrity status in the town with more hoardings and pamphlets all around Faridabad than any other film star and is busy achieving 'Ab Tak 7000' angioplasty (he claims it to be highest in Haryana). Would anybody like to help him increase the number to make it a world record, for that you may have to put your life in danger?

Among the most, the oldest, the first kind of research and awards among the cardiologists the one I find the most innovative is the "Most Profitable doctor Award "which was once won by an Indian cardiologist Dr. Prasad Chalasani at Lawnwood's Cardiac Catheterization Lab although unofficially. Today the cardiologist have become so commercial that they forget that their real goal is to cure and care of the patient and not profit. That is the reason why every now and then cardiologists are caught in scams and fraud. To consider the seriousness of the issue consider some of the recently caught frauds and scams related to angioplasty and stent industry. In February 2013 Anti Corruption Bureau (ACB) had caught Dr D. Seshagiri Rao (H.O.D Cardiac Dept. of Nizam's Insititute of Medicines (NIMS) accepting bribe of 1.6 Lakh for favoring a particular stent company. It is a trend among some cardiologist to favor some stent company for money. Some time back our honorable ex-president of India APJ Abdul Kalam had procured stent fit for commercial sale at @ Rs 10,000/- whereas commercially the range at which a stent is being sold worldwide varies between Rs 55,000 to Rs 2,50,000. Now it is understood that why the costing of stent is so high when its production cost is just a fraction of it.

The case of Dr. D. Seshagiri Rao is not only a strong case, rather a cardiologist not involved directly or indirectly in any stent/angioplasty related fraud case is rare.

To understand the seriousness of the major medical conspiracy, consider some cases.

Case 1:

1) The MCI's ethics committee found Dr. Rakesh Verma, head of department of cardiology at Safdarjung Hospital, New Delhi., guilty of unprofessional conduct in dealing with a "hapless patient". Dr. Verma was charged with indiscriminately prescribing stents for the patient and also making money from it. All the evidence produced by

the patient were serious and could not be ignored," said a member of the committee. "The MCI held at least three meeting, despite several notices the doctor ignored the hearings" he said. In July 2010, a case of disproportionate asset was registered under Prevention of Corruption Act against Dr. Verma as per the CBI's information Dr. Verma allegedly accumulated properties worth of 10 crore.

My comment: According to the government document the maximum salary of a cardiologist is about Rs 70,000/- now assuming Dr. Verma is able to save 100% of his salary then it will take him nearly 119 years to earn Rs 10 crores.

Indian Cardioligists are not only making India proud but creating an expample in other parts of the world too.

Let's take a note of few examples:

Case 2:

Dr. Mahmood Patel, M.D who has been practicing interventional cardiology in Lafayette, Louisiana and surrounding areas for more than 25 years, was falsifying patient symptoms in medical records, falsifying findings on medical tests, and performing unnecessary coronary procedures such as deploying angioplasty balloon and stents. Testimony from experts in cardiology specialist revealed that the defendant deployed stents, balloons and radiation in coronary arteries that had little or insignificant diseases. Dr. Patel faces a maximum of ten years imprisonment, a fine not more than $250,000.00 and a term of not more than three years of supervised release following confinement.

Case 3:

In February 2013 more than 400 patients sued St. Joseph Hospital in London, Kentucky. Dr. Sandesh Patil of Kentucky Medical Centre was found to implant stent unnecessary in three out of 5 patients whose records were examined.

Case 4:

In 2009 cardiologist Dr Vidya Banka of Pennsylvania Hospital had to resign as a result of allegation of unnecessarily implantation of stents. This is not just limited to Indian Cardiologists, the same is true for many other cardiologists world over.

Case 5:

In 10 April 2013, Dr Jose Katz pleaded guilty to falsifying charts, diagnosing patients with angina and other heart ailments so he could prescribe extra tests and treatments when 100's of patients did not need them. It was known to be the largest fraud by a single doctor in New York.

Case 6:

In 2011, nine Italian cardiologists were arrested in broad investigation of research fraud and misconduct for performing unauthorized clinical trial involving stent and angioplasty.

Case 7:

In November 2011, John Mclean. M.D, a cardiologist in Salisbury, Maryland was sentenced to 97 months in prison followed by three years of supervised release as a result of his conviction of fraud in connection with his submission of insurance claims for inserting unnecessary cardiac stents.

After going through the above case it, would not be a surprise for you to relate that these days salespeople for the stent making companies are allowed inside cardiac department run a violation of hospital rules and patient privacy.

I had several encounters with cardiologists during my writing of this book, and during my interaction with a celebrated white collared cardiologist when I posed a question that why the cardiologists don't treat the patient with nutrition and life style modification methods (as discussed in the book) rather than putting stents or going for angioplasty. The cardiologist on the condition of anonymity said that "If I perform angioplasty or bypass surgery I will get at least Rs 4 to 5 lakh (majorly from insurance company) but if I spend that time teaching the nutrition method to clean the blockage and reverse a heart disease the insurance company will pay not more than Rs 5,000/-. No surprise that in India multi crore stent industry is witnessing an annual growth of 25% with staggering 3 lakh stents consumed annually.

Now it may not be surprising for you to know that a report published in The Economic Times (Aug 3, 2013) says that Kerala is the state with least number of doctors (1.1 doctors per 1000 patients) and the life expectancy in Kerala is highest.

On the other hand Haryana is the state with most number of doctors (2.4 doctors per 1000 patients) and Haryana is the state with the most number of sick people.

Similarly, Doctor-Patient relation can be sensed through an interesting article published in British Medical Journal "Mortality rate drops when doctors go on strike." Now it is an open secret and it is more clear from the cover article of 'August 2011 Newsweek' issue with an article named "The One Word that Can Save Your Life: NO (to Modern Medicines)!"

The conduct these days of the cardiologists remind me of a cartoon "cardiac surgeon and a robber" by a small kid and hidden behind his innocence is the truth of cardiac surgeons.

SIMILARITIES BETWEEN CARDIAC SURGEON AND A ROBBER

Robber	Cardiac surgeon
Robber wears a mask	Doctor wears a face mask
They always threatens or force you to fulfill their demands.	They always threatens or force you to fulfill their demands

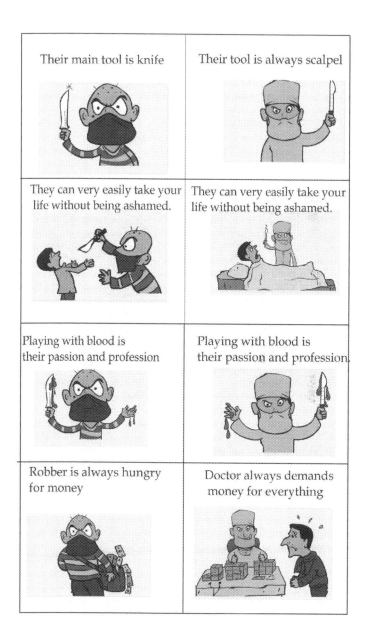

Their main tool is knife

Their tool is always scalpel

They can very easily take your life without being ashamed.

They can very easily take your life without being ashamed.

Playing with blood is their passion and profession

Playing with blood is their passion and profession.

Robber is always hungry for money

Doctor always demands money for everything

On one side most of the cardiologists are engaged in profit making out of very injurious and often life threatening surgeries. On the other hand there are doctors who are selflessly popularizing the lifestyle based methods to treat heart disease. Foremost among them is my mentor Dr T. Colin Campbell and his colleagues, Dr. Caldwell Esselstyn (batch mate of the inventor of bypass, surgeon Dr. René Gerónimo Favaloro).

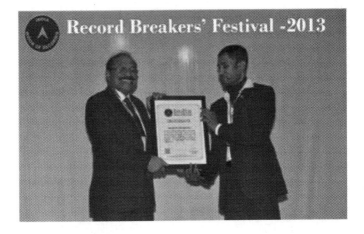

In India Dr. Bimal Chajjer once a cardiac physician with AllMS realized very early in his career that the procedure which he learnt in his M.D are not needed by the humanity and resigned from AIIMS (as well as from surgery profession) and started a chain of Heart Centre with a name Saaol Heart Centre (New Delhi) with as many as 25 centres internationally. He pioneered in India the concept that most of the heart blockages can be treated just by a Diet Modification and Nutrition Based Lifestyle Changes

Similarly another cardiologist Dr. Pratiksha Gandhi of Mumbai has taken the courageous step of discarding the high profit profession of bypass surgery and angioplasty and benefitted thousands of patients through her simple life style method (similar to the one given in the book) to reverse heart disease. She is the founder and chairperson of IPC Heart Care Centre.

One of my doctor friends, Dr Mahender Kabra, who has been practicing for last 4 decades, for the patients and not for profit and is credited with writing, curing thousands of patients (including reversing the heart blockage of his wife Dr Mamta Kabra) the natural way without involving complicated and life threatening surgeries. I once asked why there are not many doctors practicing for the benefit of patients rather than benefit of business, he said that the problem with medical industry is that if you practice something away from the protocol taught by the industry then you will be seen with hostility.

Of course it take a lot of courage to do what is right even if it means that you will be seen as a rebel. At least one more doctor Iwish I could name in the category of T. Colin Campbell or Dr. Bimal Chajjer is Dr. Devi Shetty of Narayan Hrudayalaya. Personally I respect him for his dedication for working towards reducing the cost of cardiac surgery by at least 50 %. But my point is had he worked in line of Dr T.Colin and Dr. Caldwell Esselstyn i.e cure through Diet Modification Methods (as in the book) then patient literally did not have to spend penny to reverse a heart disease and that way he could save India's losing economy. According to the recent report by Harvard School of Public Health India looses (an average) Rs 224687000 crore every year equivalent to 18.8 % of GDP due to non-communicable diseases (NCD) like heart diseases, diabetes and High Blood Pressure. These diseases affect the person in their productive years. They reduce productivity and lead to early retirement. Also they put immense pressure on public health expenditure as in most cases the treatment costs are higher compared to communicable diseases.

The thing that motivated me the most in writing this book is the result I got in my clinic in Faridabad and result produced during my health workshops. Some of the results you will find in the next few pages of the book. I understand this chapter spills the beans of some of the prestigious cardiologists which may not be taken in positive sense. I propose an open debate with any of the cardiologists named in this book or any other cardiac doctor for that matter. I also propose to initiate an investigation of the records of the tests prescribed by hospitals, of the patients who underwent bypass surgery or angioplasty in last 5 years if I am proven wrong I am ready to face the consequences.

How to get started?

If you share the same concern as mine, then you can join the movement of educating the people to become their own doctor and save themselves from diseases and doctors.

For consultancy or professional certification program please call us at,

Dr. Biswaroop Roy Chowdhury
Mob no- +91-9312286540

Chapter 8

Science of Mind—
Beyond Medical Science

In this chapter we would like to tell you about the mistakes that are being made by our cardiologists. During their treatment, which step is it that they are forgetting as a result of which the disease presents itself in its hideous form? In actuality, they treat our body, but forget that the mind also needs to be treated along with the body. By merely treating the physical ailments or symptoms alone, the body doesn't attain complete well being. Here the coordination between the heart and brain is of great importance. If the body is to be kept in a good condition, it is essential to concentrate on the well being of the mind as well.

Medicines are only a part of any treatment, and our brain and mind play their respective roles too in this process. We shall give you an example to illustrate how our mind perceives things.

Many people are scared of cockroaches despite being aware that it is harmless creature. They start shouting on seeing it. Why are those people scared of it? When asked this question, they are not able to give a valid reply. In actuality, this has a connection with the mental image they have made of this creature. When a child sees a cockroach for the first time he doesn't have fear or particular attraction towards it. Just to keep him away, the parents tell, "Go back, this is a ghost." Now, this child who has listened to abundant stories about ghosts has never seen one in reality and hence believes the cockroach to be a ghost. After this, whenever the word ghost comes up, the picture of a cockroach emerges in the child's mind. Thus, the bond between a ghost and a cockroach becomes so strong that it becomes the second name for fear. Now, after many years when he sees the cockroach, his mind asks him to feel scared because from childhood the cockroach had been connected to the fear of a ghost.

Now we'll have to see how the brain works. At first it works with its own intellect and then it makes use of its stored up memory. If it has to choose between the two, it chooses the mental pictures stored from childhood. Before understanding or agreeing with any argument, it takes the help of its past memories. Only if when these memories give their consent, the brain agrees to it.

If we need to put something into our brain, we have to input something that is related to it and only then will it accept the change. Let us assume that a person is going to run a 100 metre race. At present he is practising for the race. Even before he starts to run and the reverse counting begins, his heart starts to beat fast. Though this person doesn't have to face any challenge or doesn't need any energy, yet his brain and heart are in conversation. They are aware that this particular person's body under goes such changes whenever he has to run. This is a result of his practise. Using this person's previous experience and from the memory stored, the brain decides that it has to make this person win in this race. Now when this person begins to run, his brain is aware that at that moment the digestive system doesn't need energy to digest food and it diverts most of the energy for the activity of running. By running the person's body temperature increases and in order to protect the body from any loss due to this rise the brain activates the sweat glands. When the person sweats, the body temperature reduces automatically. The person keeps running and the brain knows that he would need water. Normally when we drink lots of water, we need to urinate after a while. But here, the brain knows that the person cannot stop anywhere. Hence, no matter how much water he drinks he will not have the desire to urinate. All the means or the mediums that are needed to aid the completion of his aim are already set in his brain.

Now we should know the value of emotions in our life. Let's have a look at the picture below:

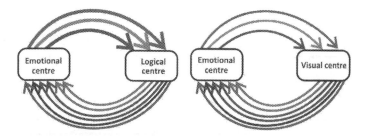

motions control logic and logic controls emotions, but emotions have a greater influence. Our emotions are also influenced by the visual centre. As a result, the logical power is also influenced.

Heart-Brain connection:

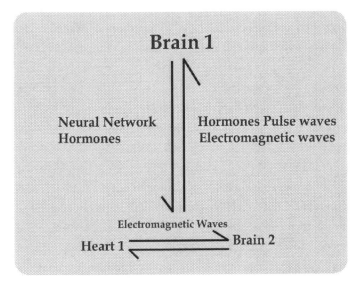

If the brain wants to convey something to the heart, it makes use of the neural network and hormones, and similarly, if the heart wants to convey something to the brain, it makes use of the pulse wave, hormones and electromagnetic waves. These waves play an important role in this connection.

Consider that you are going to your friend's house. The door opens after it is knocked for a while. The friend welcomes you with a smile, seats you in a room and goes inside to get something. Though there was no shortcoming in your welcome, you feel restless. Actually, just before your arrival there, there had been an argument between the husband and wife regarding something, which stopped on hearing the knock on the door. What you are experiencing at this moment is because of the heart's electromagnetic waves. They are leaving their influence on the surrounding environment, which has been absorbed by your heart. Even without knowing anything, you sensed the restlessness that had spread in the surroundings.

You meet a person for the first time and get a feeling of oneness. You meet some other person for the first time and after meeting him, you don't feel at ease. You say that he is not compatible with you. Actually, this is because of the electromagnetic waves released by the heart. Though our brain also releases electromagnetic waves, the waves sent by the heart are 500 times more powerful.

If we feel that we must leave a positive stamp by not only our verbal communication, but also by our non-verbal communication, and that the person in front of us behaves in the manner we want him to, then we have to concentrate on the electromagnetic waves sent out by our heart. We have to control them. But first lets see how all this happens? We must understand the fact that our electromagnetic waves and of the person in front of us mutually influence each other. The outflow of our words has only partial impact. This means that when we talk to someone, he is definitely influenced by the words that we say, but also our body language at that time, the feelings towards that person in our mind and the waves emanating have no lesser importance.

Take a look at the figure below to see blow how the consensus and contradiction of the heart and brain show their effect:

```
┌─ Positive feelings ◄┐  ┌─ Negative feelings ◄┐
│                     │  │                      │
│                     │  │                      │
└►Heart-Brain consensus ─┘  └►Heart-Brain contradiction ─┘
```

The person who has positive feelings always has a mind filled with happiness and positivity, but around the person who always has negative feelings, a negative environment is formed. He gets tangled in that environment and lives in it. He searches for negativity and hopelessness in each and every action of his. Here the consensus between the heart and brain is same as that in discordant music. When all and move ahead, then many actions will automatically take place with ease.

Research has revealed that the following results can exhibit due to unhealthy feelings:

- Incapability to think clearly
- Lesser decision making capacity
- Lesser physical coordination
- Increase in chances of heart diseases
- Chances of increased blood pressure (hypertension)

"In more than half of the cases related to heart diseases, It has been found that factors like high cholesterol, smoking or sedentary life style have not been found responsible."

-Integrative Physiological and Behavioural Science

We suddenly hear of a healthy person dying due to heart problem. There were no risk factors in his life. These happened due to the incompatibility of the heart and brain. Due to this lack of harmony life seems empty and burdensome.

According to a report by the University of London, a person who is highly tense and has negative thoughts is six times more at the risk of dying due to cancer and heart diseases as compared to a person who smokes ten cigarettes a day.

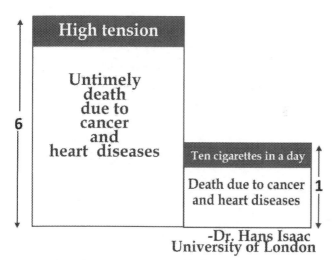

"The result of a ten year study shows that when compared to smoking, death due to cancer and heart diseases due to stress and tension has been more. A person who does not take considerable steps to reduce tension has a 40% greater chance of dying when compared to a person who is not tense."

-British Journal of Medical Psychology

IN a report published in the British Medical Journal about a research on approximately ten thousand Government officials. These were the employees who were in constant fear of losing their job and they were compared with those employees who were living with safe jobs and it was found that in comparison with those who held a secure post, the rate of coronary heart problems was double in these people.

-British Medical Journal (1988)

The Harvard Medical School conducted a research on 1623 such people who had survived a heart attack. It was found that when these people lost their temper in an emotional situation, they were at a double risk of having a heart attack when compared to those who remained calm.

What is our life? The shaded region in the picture depicts our life. Our life is made up of a mixture of our mind, environment and body. When a doctor treats a person he only works on the body. We have to work on all the three-mind, body and environment. Let's assume

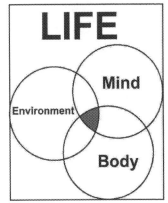

that we have to appear for an examination. At this time if we have a good relationship between our heart and brain, giving the examination will be easy. I am not saying that you will know the answers to the questions that you have not learnt, but it is sure you will be able to give the answers to the questions you have learnt in the correct manner. On coming out of the examination hall you will not have the grievance that despite preparing well you were able to answer only a few questions.

On achieving a proper connection between the heart and brain, or mind and brain, we will be able to have a proper balance of the mind, body and environment. In the absence of a balance no work can be completed properly. Harmony provides speed to our work. When we do a job which we like, the brain and heart beat rhythmically. The outcome of such a work is always good, but we don't get to do the work of our choice often. In such a case what stance should we take? Before commencing any work, we should bring about coordination between our heart and brain.

Now, through a picture we would like to show what role is played by the immune system of the body.

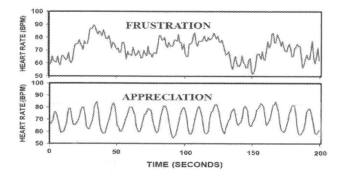

It has been shown in this picture that when a person loses his temper his immunity towards diseases increases suddenly and then drops to the lowest point. On the other hand when there is someone to take care of or to shower love, the capacity to fight diseases increases little, then drops little and then slowly begins to increase. It is clear from this that our immunity also changes with each beat of the heart. Here too everything is dependent on the coordination between the heart and brain.

You have learnt about the electromagnetic waves that are released from the heart. With these waves as a medium an electromagnetic region in formed. Just as there is magnetic energy between two magnets, so is there an electromagnetic region between two people. Let us assume that you go to meet a known person, but after meeting him you feel there was something wrong in his behaviour. He had not behaved in the manner he should have. If we go to the root of this we may tell that there is some mistake on your part too. When you stepped into his office you were not convinced about his behaviour. Due to the electromagnetic waves that came from your heart, he had started to feel restless and did not behave in the manner he should have behaved with you.

Let me also tell you that when we meet a person for the first time the touch of our hands are also of importance. You can understand this well with the help of the graph shown in next page.:

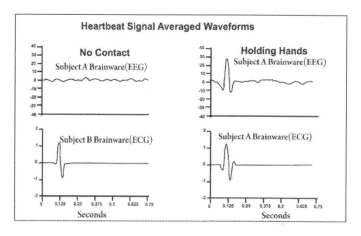

It has been shown that when two people meet their electromagnetic waves get attracted mutually. In the second part of the graph we have shown what happened after the two people shook hands after meeting. The EEG of a person's brain and the ECG of the other person's heart were taken and the presence of equality in their model was noted. Both had attracted each other to some extent.

Heartbeat Signal Averaged Waveforms

To substantiate this, the article published in the New England Journal of Medicine, February 1996 can be taken into account, in which it has been mentioned that after the earthquake at the North Bridge, Los Angeles, there was a sudden increase in deaths due to heart attack. Even though the people in the neighbouring areas were safe from the earthquake, but their hearts were affected by the news of the deaths taking place due to the earthquake in their surrounding areas.

"During the first Gulf war, it has been found in the Israeli hospitals that there has been a sudden increase in deaths owing to heart attacks."

-September 1991—The Lancet

"As a result of post traumatic stress disorder after the September 11, 2001 terrorist attack, many people have lost their lives."

-March 2002, New England Journal of Medicine

Many of those who died due to this, included people who neither were involved directly in the attack nor were their families involved, but were mere witness to the event. The dreadfulness of the incident caused severe stress thus resulting in death.

I want to mention here that due to our negative thoughts and attitude, the harmony between the heart and brain is disrupted, while positive thoughts create harmony between the heart and brain. We can understand the difference between the two from the following picture:

Positive thoughts	**Negative thoughts**
⬇	⬇
Harmony between heart and brain	Disharmony between heart and brain
⬇	⬇
1. Increase in oxytocin (love hormone)	1. Increase in cortisol (stress hormone)
2. Increase in production of white blood cells	2. Decrease in white blood cell production

3. Colon getting emptied	3. Colon not getting cleansed
4. Emptying of urinary bladder	4. Time taken to empty urinary bladder
5. Increase in energy inflow into body.	5. Decrease in energy inflow into body.
6. Increase in digestive enzymes	6. Decrease in digestive enzymes.
7. Secretion of saliva in mouth	7. Drying of Saliva in mouth

Thought process of the brain

Our brain often shows us only what we want to see. Prior to the commencement of a job we form an opinion about the job which is based on our previous experiences. After that all our work rests on these thoughts.

Our brain always brings our past experiences into work. For instance, if a patient's hand is cut off, even after a while after the surgery, he complains of itching in the part which has been cut off. This is considered a psychological problem, but our brain also has a part to play in it. The patient's brain has not yet accepted the fact that a part has been cut off, hence by creating a desire to scratch the part, it consoles itself that the part is still in the body. Due to its past experiences it keeps making such commiserations.

Our heart ensures that there is proper blood supply throughout the body. God has provided a few hidden arteries to keep this machine working. These arteries are known as collateral arteries. When the original arteries stop working, the brain and heart together get these hidden arteries to work. To understand this let us take the example of a vehicle which has a stepney. If the vehicle gets punctured, the help of the stepney can be taken. But to get this done, the vehicle has to be stopped and someone's help is to be taken as we cannot fix the puncture of a tyre in a moving vehicle. Similarly, a proper harmony between the brain and heart has to be made in order to activate the hidden arteries when it is needed.

There are more than 1.5 crore heart patients in India. Among the heart patients in the world, sixty percent are Indians. The remaining forty percent are from the rest of the world. One third of the deaths in the entire world are due to heart diseases. The option of activating the collateral arteries is available with the brain, but this is possible only if there is perfect harmony between the heart and the brain. This is not an imagination or a mere thought. In actuality, we can bring about this change in our brain within two days.

We can see these arteries in our heart but cannot bring them into use. The technique to do so has a great connection with our heart and brain. It often happens that during times of emergency we have a good connection between the heart and brain and are able to achieve good results.

Recollect the incident of the itching in the cut off part. When the patient repeatedly talks of the itching in the cut off part the doctor takes the help of the past experiences of the brain. He asks the patient to close his eyes and imagine that he is scratching the part that has been cut off. The patient scratches the part in his imagination and then he gets satisfaction.

These examples show us that man is not just the body and in any disease it is not enough to just get the body treated. We have to go beyond the body and treat the mind and heart as well. The surprising fact is that medical education does not teach this relationship between the body and the mind. There is no place for this topic in their curriculum.

Chapter 9

My Experiments with Truth

Friends, just imagine that you just heard an announcement about the invention of a new car which can repair itself on its own, I mean once the car broke down, you leave the car for a while and it will get repaired automatically. If it gets punctured, within few a minutes it will get repaired magically. If there is some wear and tear in the engine's piston, you don't need the intervention of mechanic. Just wait and it will get back to the original condition in some days. It can happen only in fantasy. But the good news is that we already possess that amazing vehicle. That is the human body. Human body has immense spare capacity to come back to its original form. No matter whatever is your physical condition at this moment. Whether you are suffering from a heart disease or cancer or kidney failure. You can heal yourself, that too without any artificial modern medicinal/surgical intervention. Rather trying to heal with medicine/surgery which makes the situation even more complicated and worse.

You just have to give your body the right condition (as given in the book), right environment including food and rest. Given the kind of mental state, the body starts the process of reversing a disease. Based on this science of body, I conducted health workshops worldwide including U.A.E, Kuwait, Vietnam, Abu Dhabi, Nepal and India and have covered more than 100 cities. It worked every time at every place for everybody. Here are some of the testimonials of the participants who joined my health workshop as well as patients who visited me at my Faridabad Clinic last year (2013).

Special Comments of Patients of Faridabad Clinic
City: Faridabad   Venue: Faridabad Clinic
Date: 15 April 2013 to 31 December 2013

"Now I feel less constipated, less irritataled & more active".
-Rohan, Student

"I have much relief in pain."
-Rohit Kumar, Teacher

"My dose was reduced to half after first week of onset of treatment."
-Master Aryan student, Student

"I feel light, there is improvement in hormonal levels."
-Ms Ruhina, Homemaker

"My TLC level is reduced."
-Rattan Singh, Service

"I had cyst in ovary but now I don't require medicine now after following "The China Study Diet Plan".

-Ms Tanu, Homemaker

"My weight is reduced & no swelling in my feet."

-Ms Pinki Sharma, Student

"No more swelling in my body and a relief in pain."

-Ms Rano Devi, Homemaker

"My cholesterol level is reduced."

-Mr Sushil Chand, Yoga Teacher

"I got relief in pain and reduction in gastritis."

-Mr P.K Sharma, Businessman

"Much Improvement in dryness of my mouth."

-Ms Ritu Sharma, Student

"Me and my doctor is feeling much improvement in my health condition."

-Ms. Kruti Nagpal, Homemaker

"I got a relief in back pain."

-Ms Shruti Singh, Teacher

"My BP now remains normal & doctor has cut down my medication."

-Mr Manav Panday, Govt. Serviceman

"Now I have sound sleep and no stress."

-Mr Jagmohan Singh, Serviceman

"I have very less inflammation and no pain."

-Ms Ritu Gupta, Homemaker

"Now I have no depression and feel less irritated."

-Mr Lakshit Jain, Businessman

"There is a lot of improvement in my problem of piles."

-Mr JK Singh, Serviceman

"I lost two kg weight in 3 months after having this special diet."

-Mr Ramesh, Businessman

"I am feeling 75% improvement in gastritis problem."

-Ms Sunita, Homemaker

"I got benefit from stomach pain as well as chest pain after consuming China Study Diet Plan."

-Abhimanyu Kushwaha, Businessman

"I have a relief from gas trouble."

-Shankar Lal Verma, Businessman

"My weight is reduced from 91.8 kg to 84kg after implementing The China Study Diet Plan."

-Shorya Singh, Social Worker

"My health is improved a lot and stamina is increased after following The China Study Diet Plan."

-Sh B.S Bajaj, Businessman

"By consuming Raw Food on daily basis my constipation problem is diminished now."

-Gagan Kumar, Serviceman

"There is a lot of improvement in cervical pain and have a great relief."

-Abhay Kumar Jha, Businessman

"My diabetic problem is in control after following The China Study Diet Plan."

-Poonam, Homemaker

"Feeling energetic and now body pain is quite less."

-K. Baghel, Serviceman

"I have a relief in constipation and moreover had a pain on one ride of chest which is now reduced."

-Naresh Dalal, Govt. Teacher

"Feeling light, and have confidence now to cure renal failure with Raw Food Diet Plan."

-Vinod Kumar Mittal, Businessman

"I got relief in acidity and feeling more energetic and light."

-Vikkrant Singh, Serviceman

"I had high cholesterol, after following China Study Diet Plan, feeling light and energetic."

-Parminder Singh, Businessman

"I was suffering from diabetes, this special Diet Plan has improved my health a lot."

-Poonam, Teacher

"This diet has provided me a relief in cervical pain."

-Abhay Kumar Jha, Teacher

"I am feeling energetic and light."

-Radhika, Homemaker

Medical Report
Title: Mind, Body & Health Workshop
Organizer: Haryana State Govt. Education Department
Speaker: Dr. Biswaroop Roy Chowdhury

Number of teachers as Participants: 250
Date: From 27 April to 1 May 2013
Time: Morning 10 am to 3 pm
Place: Exhibition cum Conventional Centre, Huda Parisar, Sector-12, Faridabad

---

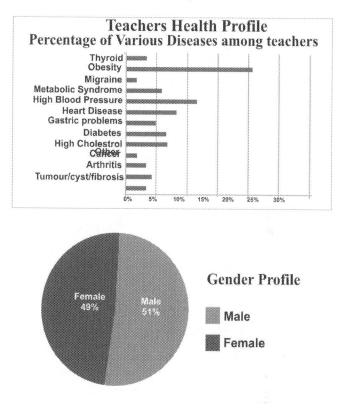

Medical Report

Title: Mind, Body & Health Workshop
Organizer: Haryana State Govt. Education Department
Speaker: Dr. Biswaroop Roy Chowdhury

Number of teachers as Participants: 250
Date: From 27 April to 1 May 2013
Time: Morning 10 am to 3 pm
Place: Exhibition cum Conventional Centre, Huda
Parisar, Sector-12, Faridabad

Feedback immediately after the Training (May 1, 2013)

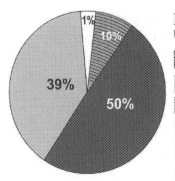

How do you rate the program

- Bad program
- Good program
- Excellent program
- One of the best program
- Best program of my life
- Just o.k (0%)

How do you rate the trainer

- Bad trainer
- Good trainer
- Excellent trainer
- One of the best trainer
- Best trainer of my life
- Just o.k (0%)

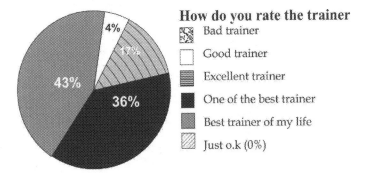

Medical Report

Title: Mind, Body & Health Workshop
Organizer: Haryana State Govt. Education Department
Speaker: Dr. Biswaroop Roy Chowdhury

Number of teachers as Participants: 250
Date: From 27 April to 1 May 2013
Time: Morning 10 am to 3 pm
Place: Exhibition cum Conventional Centre, Huda Parisar, Sector-12, Faridabad

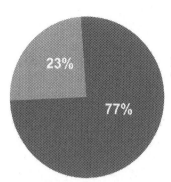

**Percentage of the Follower of
The China Study Diet Plan**

■ Followed

■ Not Followed

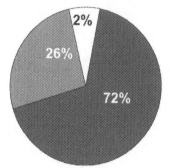

Health Profile

■ Excellent Improvement

■ Satisfactory improvement

☐ No Sign of Improvement

▨ Deterioration in Health(0%)

Health Condition of Haryana Govt. Teachers after following China Study Diet Plan for 1 month (2nd May to 2nd June 2013)

"My high BP, diabetes and sleeplessness got cured"
-Bimla Rani, Govt Primary School, Faridabad

"My wife had migraine and now she is fine"
-Moti Lal, Govt. Primary School, Jasana

"One of my colleagues showed improvement in breast cancer and I got cured from headache"
-Poonam, Govt. Girls Middle School, Chandawali

"My thyroid level is under control and my weight has also reduced"

-Manju, Govt. Middle School Bijopur

"My cholesterol level is under control and now I am not taking any medicine"

-Anil kumar, Govt. Primary School, Faridabad

"After taking this diet my BP and diabetes got controlled and doctor reduced the dose of my medicine"

-Vinay Kumar, Govt. School, Faridabad

"I lost 6kgs weight in a month"

-Rekha, Govt. Middle School Badrola

"I got relief from pain in legs and bones"

-Shashi, Govt. High School Indra Nagar Faridabad

"My digestion improved greatly"

-Nem Singh, Govt. Middle School, Nangla Jogiyan

"I got relief from constant pain in feet"

-Murti Devi, Govt. Middle School, Sec-10, Faridabad

"My constipation is gone and my colleague's thyroid levels are under control"

-Indu Wadhwa, Govt. Boys High School No.2,
NIT Faridabad

"I got relief from cough"

-Pitamber, Govt. Primary School, Pakhal

"I lost 4 kgs just by taking raw food and now feel very energetic"

-Narender, Govt. School, Faridabad

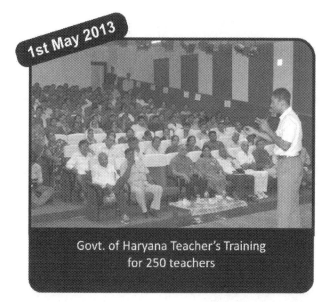

Govt. of Haryana Teacher's Training
for 250 teachers

Thanks to Ms. Sunaina Ranjan (Principal Secretory Haryana Govt) for making this project successful.

Medical Report
Title: Mind, Body & Health Workshop
Organizer: Indian Army
Speaker: Dr. Biswaroop Roy Chowdhury

Number of Participants: 180
Date: From 8 May to 10 May 2013
Time: Morning 10 am to 3 pm
Place: Army Auditorium, Port Blair

Army Personnel Profile

Percentage of Various Diseases among Army Personnel

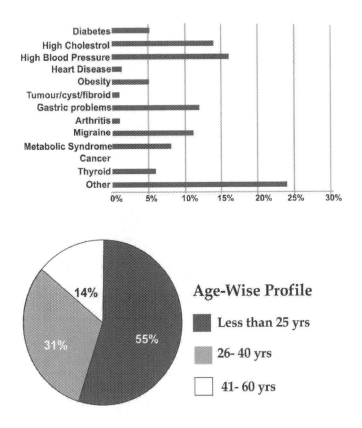

Feedback immediately after the Training (10 May-13)

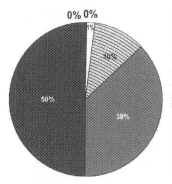

How do you rate the program

▨ Bad program
☐ Good program
▤ Excellent program
■ One of the best program
▨ Best program of my life
▨ Just o.k (0%)

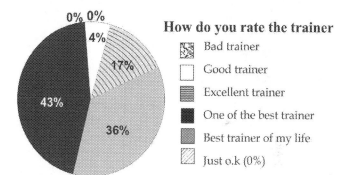

How do you rate the trainer

▨ Bad trainer
☐ Good trainer
▤ Excellent trainer
■ One of the best trainer
▨ Best trainer of my life
▨ Just o.k (0%)

Medical Report

Title: Mind, Body & Health Workshop
Organizer: Indian Army
Speaker: Dr. Biswaroop Roy Chowdhury

Number of Participants: 180
Date: From 8 May to 10 May 2013
Time: Morning 10 am to 3 pm
Place: Army Auditorium, Port Blair

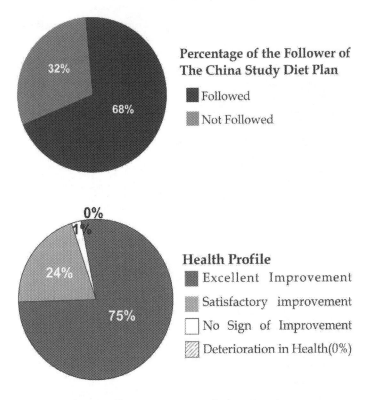

Percentage of army personnel showing improvement in Diabetes, High Cholesterol, High BP, Heart Diseases, Obesity, Cancer, Cyst, Fibroid, Gastric, Arthritis, Migraine, Metabolic Syndrome, Thyroid and other lifestyle related diseases.

Health Condition of Indian Army Personnel in Portblair after following China Study Diet Plan for 1 month (10th May to 10 June 2013)

"My blood pressure dropped down to normal after this diet"
-Surinder Kumar, Portblair

"My stomach is getting properly cleansed and there's Increase in my energy level"
-Havildar Charanjeet Singh Portblair

"My chest pain got cured, after I started this diet"
-Sukhwinder Singh, Portblair

"There's great improvement in my digestion and related gastric problems"

-Jasvir singh

"No more pain in my legs and my energy level has also increased"

-Havildar Sridhar Ch

"The bulky feeling after the meals has been replaced with light and I recommended it to others too"
-Havildar Sreejith

"I wake up feeling fresh in the morning"
-EDN Clk Rakesh Jakhar

"I feel fresh all the time ever since I started consuming raw diet"

-Subedar Bikar singh

"My acidity reduced since I started this diet"

-22 Punjab Regiment Iqbal singh

"I started feeling energetic"

-Satyvir Singh

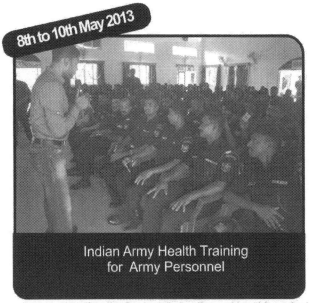

Thanks to Brigadier Sanjay Thakur for making this project successful.

Special Comments of Participants of Health Workshop

City: VAPI   Date: 12th Jan 2013
Venue: Via House Auditorium

"Within 21 days I lost 7 kg and my son in 9th class has left junk food completely."

-Rajeev, Businessman

"I lost 7-8 kgs of weight, pain in my foot has stopped, and now I feel energetic."

-Narendra, Businessman

"Weight is under control and energy level has been increased."

-Ms Lavanya, Pshychologist

"I got permanent relief from infection in stomach which had been there since last 2 years."

-Ms Shahnaz, Housewife

"Now I feel healthy and my arthritis pain is reduced."
-Ms Arpana, Housewife

"Got relieved from asthma."
-Mr. Naik Krishna, serviceman

"I feel energetic throughout the day, I didn't suffer from cold and cough from last 6 months which was very much frequent."

-Mr Dev Kumar, Businessman

"My Health got improved and my weight got increased as I was underweight"

-Ms Farhin, Businesswoman

"My back pain is reduced, I have started feeling light and my activeness has been increased."

-Nazeer, Govt. servant, Paramedical staff

"I don't have frequent high temperature now, my son had severe constipation but now he is completely cured."

-Ms Parinita, Student

"Pimples on my face got reduced."

-Mr. Keshav, Businessman

Special Comments of Participants of Health Workshop

City: Chandigarh   Date: 27th Jan 2013

Venue: St. Stephen's School Auditorium

"I don't feel tired any more. My wife was overweight, she reduced up to 8-9kgs. Also her thyroid problem got cured within two months of having raw food. Her medication is being stopped by an allopathic doctor"

-Lalit Bishnoi, Engineer

"My B.P level had gone down and I have stopped taking medicines after following The China Study Diet Plan"

-Dr.Anoop, Teacher

"I have felt marvelous improvement in me, Raw food is panacea for every ailment, improvement in physical and mental condition, my mother was hard of hearing she had started hearing now. MYRIAD BENEFITS"

-H.S Sethi, Businessman

"My Wife was having thyroid, now she does not need any medication after following raw food plan suggested by Dr Roy"

-Jagjeet Sngh, Businessman

"My Husband got benefited in asthma through the China Study Diet Plan."

-Samita, Housewife

"I feel more energetic and more younger."

-R.K.Mahajan, Businessman

Special Comments of Participants of Health Workshop
City: Shimla   Date: 31st March-1st April 2013
Venue: Gaiety Heritage

"I am following "The China Study Diet Plan" and lost weight by 2-3 kgs in a month."

-Anshul Sharma, Student

"Now I feel energetic and light."

-Prateek Sharma, Student

"My immune system got strengthened which was very weak earlier."

-Abhinav Sharma, Student

Special Comments of Agartala Seminar
Date 25 April 2013
Venue: Nazrul Kala Kshetra Place Agartala

"I lost weight and my sugar level also got reduced."
-Dipanwita, Teacher

"I have started feeling more energetic"
-Bikas Kanti, Administration

'I have lost some weight, my gastric problem got reduced and now I feel more energetic"
-Dulal Sen, Businessman

"My cholesterol levels got reduced and liver problem is cured.
-Chandan Singha, Businessman

"My gastric problem got cured completely after taking raw food"
-Mita Saha, Housewife

"My constipation problem is gone"
-Santanu Prasad Das, Serviceman

"My thyroid hormone levels became normal and hemoglobin got increased."
-Ratna Bhattacharya, Teacher

"My problem of constipation is completely cured'
-Manilal Chakraborty, Tabla Artist

Special Comments of Participants of Health Workshop
City: Ajmer   Date: 13 May 2013
Venue: Jawahar Rang Manch

"My diabetes is cured and medicine is stopped and cholesterol levels became normal, my energy level has also increased"
                    -Chitrang Singh, Retired govt. employee

"Diabetic (sugar) levels came in normal range, and weight is reduced."
                                    -Aditya, Businessman

"I lost 5 kg in 2 months, started feeling light, my alertness increased and quality of life has improved."
                    -Ms Prafulla Vaidya, Businessman

"I remain energetic throughout the whole day."
                            -Yagya Deo, Bank Officer

"My anxiety levels and aggression has decreased."
                        -Dinesh Dutt, Businessman

"Energy level has increased, and I got relief from leg pain."
                            -Ms Renu, Housewife

"My stamina has increased, dullness and laziness has reduced."
                        -Dinesh Gupta, Retired Lecturer

Special Comments of Participants of Health Workshop
City: Almora   Venue: Hotel Shikar
Date: 23 May 2013

"Stopped taking medicine for any problem and in cold, cough or any other minor problem I take raw food and get well very soon."

-Jagdish Prasad, Teacher

"I feel light and more energetic through-out the day."

-Lalita Rautela, Teacher

"I have migraine and now frequency of headache has reduced"

-Rashmi Pandey, Teacher

"My digestion is improved, energy level has increased."

-L D Malkani, Govt. Service

Special Comments of School Principals
of Health Workshop
City: Gurgaon   Venue: SCERT Gurgaon
Date: 25 May 2013

"My digestion is improving, and Improvement in blood pressure is also felt."

-Rajmalyes, AMSSS Hasanpur

"I lost 6-7 kg of weight in 1 month."

-Mr Sunil Kumar, AMSSS Bawla Resident

"My weight was 84 kgs and now it is 79 kgs."

-Pramod, AMSSS Mandheta Resident

"I lost 2-3 kgs of my weight, and now I feel fresh, and got relief from knee pain."

-Mr Brij Bala Saini, Govt. Senior Sec School Kanheri

"I lost 3 kgs of my weight."

-Ramesh Kumar,
Aarohi Model Senior Secondary School
Nathusari Kalan

"My problem of digestion has been improved & I have lost 2 kgs of my weight."

-Mr Prem Kamboj, AMSSS, Jhiri Resident

"My digestion problem is reduced and I feel light and energetic."

-Jagjeet Singh, AMS School Kheri Surera

"No more constipation, and pain in back bone is relieved my mother had body ache now it is reduced & my father's stomach problem is cured"

-Sanjay Kumar,
Aarohi Model Senoir Secondary School,
Mohamadpuria

Special Comments of Participants of Health Workshop
City: Tadong Gangtok   Date: 20th-25th July
Venue: Sikkim Govt. College Auditorium

"My Diabetes is under control after following The China Study Diet Plan"

-Ms Anjana, Govt. Service

"My BP is under control now, and I have started feeling fresh."

-Ritu Raj, Govt. service

"I lost belly fat, feeling physically and mentally active, fatigue and lethargy has gone and feeling high positive energy."

-Ms. Sony, Teacher

"My father is following The China Study Plan and his B.P is controlled."

-Ms Priya, student

"My problem of acidity has decreased, after following raw food diet plan"

-Dileep, Teacher

"I got improvement in old cough and cold."

-Mrs Durga, Govt. service

"I was suffering from bleeding, arthritis, colitis and my condition is improving with 'The China Study Diet plan"

-Mr. Mohan, Govt. Service

"I got a relief from headache after following The China Study Diet Plan"

-Ms. Payal, House Wife

Special Comments of Participants of Health Workshop
City: Bhilwara   Date: 29 July 2013
Venue: Town Hall

"I lost considerable amount of weight, my tension level has decreased after following The China Study Diet Plan"

-Mr. Prem Singh, Businessman

"I was suffering from allergy from last 15 yrs and now it is cured in 1 month by having raw food."

-Mr Navratan, Businessman

Special Comments of Participants of Health Workshop
City: Mehboobnagar,   Date: 8 August 2013
Venue: Hotel Sindhu

"I have lost some weight, I have not measured but I can feel the change."

-Md Haneef Ahmed, Teacher

"I had mild toothache from which I got relief after taking raw food."

-Pasula Chandra Shekhar, Scientist

Feedback of people attended Health Seminar
Place: Gurgoan   Date: 15th August
Venue: Om Shanti Retreat Centre

"I had stopped taking medicine for BP from last 20 days i.e just after I started taking raw diet."

-Sashi Kant Sharma, Businessman

"I had treated one patient and his diabetes is completely reversed"

-Mahesh Chandra, Consultant

"My dose of medicine for diabetes is reduced by doctor.

-Kamlesh, Housewife

"My gastric problem is cured and I feel active now"

-Mahender Kumar Jain, Govt Officer

"My face started glowing after following "The China Study Diet" Plan and my acidity problem is also cured."

-Sunita Singhal, House Wife

Special Comments of Participants of Health Workshop
City: Lucknow   Date: 24 November 2013
Venue: Sangeet Natak Academy, Gomti Nagar

"I follow "The China Study Diet "Plan everyday and feel energetic, light and bloating is no more after having lunch."

-Bharti Gandhi, Founder, City Montessori School

"My blood pressure is normal after following "The China Study Diet Plan"

-Asthma, Housewife

"I lost extra weight after adopting raw food diet."

-Arun Kumar Singh

"I don't feel bloated after having lunch and diabetes medicine dose is decreased."

-Gurmail Singh Dhillon, Businessman

"My diabetes is in control and medication is decreased."

-Omkar Verma, Serviceman

"Weight is reduced and I am quite energetic and energy level is increased"

-Piyush K Mishra, Businessman

"I have found an improvement in my overall health."

-Dr. P C Gupta, Doctor

"My health is improved after following raw food diet, feel energetic."

-Vishwas Kumar, Serviceman

"I feel energetic and light after having raw food and moreover my sugar level is also gone down."

-Tanu Shree Gupta, House wife

"I feel energetic and weakness is decreased a lot."

-Chanchal, Homemaker

"I feel energetic and healthy after having raw food."

-Vandana Gupta, Teacher

"My blood sugar level reduced down from 300mg/dL to 150mg/dL within three days"

-Mr Praful Kumar Gupta
Inspector (U.P Police)

Stop Press

1 November 2013, I was engrossed in last and final phase of editing this book. Suddenly I overhear my receptionist calling out a familiar name while conversing on a phone. "Are you Neelam Sood's Daughter "? She was asking the other person on phone. Neelam is one of the participants who attended my Health Workshop in Chandigarh held on 30th January-2013.

Speaking of her medical condition; she was in the final stage of cancer as declared by Dr. Rajiv Vedi of Fortis Hospital, Mohali. In 2009 she was initially diagnosed with breast cancer that later on metastasized to lungs, liver, bones, backbones and whole body. Doctors had failed miserably to control the spread of the cancer.

Before I could anticipate her present condition after 8 months of attending my health workshop (when doctors at the Mohali Hospital refused any further treatment), I saw a gleam of excitement and relief on receptionist's face. The news was, that doctors were not only baffled with her miraculous recovery in the last 8 months but were also wondering about her quick recovery!

Neelam underwent 8 cycles of chemotherapy from December-2012 to May-2013 but there was little improvement in her condition. Meanwhile she also started with 'The China Study Diet Plan' and discarded some of the medicines in spite of repeated insistence by the doctors to continue the medicines. After Chemotherapy she strictly followed The China Study Diet Plan "from June 2013 onwards and finally now her CT scan reports showed a 95% improvement in her cancerous liver and doctors were amazed to see the reports.

Receiving such self-satisfying news is a routine affair in my office and this is the source of courage and motivation which helps me to stand against the corrupt medical system. I am closing the book with the hope to receive your success stories and blessings which will give me strength to complete my next book in the series.

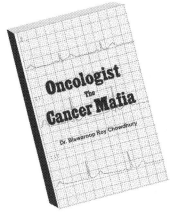

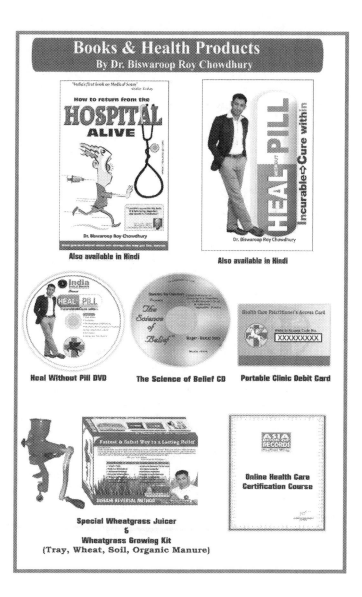

Books & Health Products
By Dr. Biswaroop Roy Chowdhury

Also available in Hindi

Also available in Hindi

Heal Without Pill DVD

The Science of Belief CD

Portable Clinic Debit Card

Special Wheatgrass Juicer
&
Wheatgrass Growing Kit
(Tray, Wheat, Soil, Organic Manure)

Online Health Care
Certification Course

WORLD RECORDS UNIVERSITY

World Records University is an autonomous university formed by the conglomeration of National Record Books all across the globe. It has its registered office in UK and India (Faridabad, Haryana).

World Records University has launched an Honorary Doctorate in Nature Science and Medicine in India with content based on Cornell University USA and Mint Culinary School, Vietnam.

Honorary Doctorate in Nature Science and Medicine:

Eligibility Criteria:

World Records University Invites applications for Honorary Doctorate from health practitioners practicing in the following fields:

- Allopathy
- Ayurveda
- Naturopathy
- Homeopathy
- Acupressure
- Acupuncture
- Physiotherapy
- Yoga
- Psychoneurobics
- Unani
- Chromotherapy
- Aromatherapy
- Magnet Therapy
- Reiki
- Neuro Linguistic Planning
- Osteopathy
- Pranic Healing
- Reflexology
- Siddha Medicine
- Qi

Steps to claim your Honorary Doctorate in Nature Science and Medicine:

Step 1: The applicant has to pass an online screening test(in Hindi, English, Vietnamese, Nepali) conducted by World Records University.

Step 2: You will be given an online study material.

Step 3: Submit doctorate application form (DAF) on the basis of your understanding of the study material (provided by World Records University).

Step 4: Write thesis on the basis of the format provided by World Records University.

Step 5: Submit your thesis.

Step 6: World Records University will authenticate the originality of your thesis and on acceptance by the panel of experts World Records University will confer you the Honorary Doctorate.

Step 7: Your thesis will be published in World Records University's annual publication.

For details contact us at www.worldrecordsuniversity.co.uk
E-mail: info@worldrecordsuniversity.com, Phone:+91-129-2510534, +91-9313378451

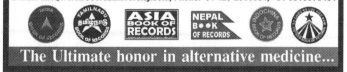

The Ultimate honor in alternative medicine...